The
Enigma
of
Health

T0219475

The
Enigma
of
Health

*The Art of Healing
in a Scientific Age*

Hans-Georg Gadamer

Translated by
Jason Gaiger and Nicholas Walker

Polity Press

This English translation: chapter 1 copyright © *Social Research* 1977;
all other chapters © Polity Press 1996. First published in German
as *Über die Verborgenheit der Gesundheit* copyright © Suhrkamp Verlag, 1993.
This translation first published by Polity Press in association with Blackwell
Publishers Ltd, 1996.

Published with the financial support of Inter Nationes, Bonn.

Reprinted 2004

Polity Press
65 Bridge Street
Cambridge, CB2 1UR, UK

Polity Press
350 Main Street
Malden, MA 02148, USA

ISBN 0-7456-1367-5
ISBN 0-7456-1594-5 (pbk)

A CIP catalogue record for this book is available from the British Library.

Typeset in Sabon 11/13pt
by Graphicraft Typesetters Ltd., Hong Kong
Printed and bound in Great Britain by Marston Book Services Limited, Oxford

This book is printed on acid-free paper.

For more information on Polity visit our website:www.polity.co.uk

Contents

Preface

It has always been a particular occasion that has prompted me to speak about problems of health care and the art of medicine. The results are gathered together in this small volume. It should not be a cause for surprise if a philosopher who is neither a doctor nor feels himself to be a patient nevertheless wishes to participate in the discussion concerning the broad range of problems which arise in the field of health in the scientific and technological age. Nowhere else do the advances of modern research enter so directly into the sociopolitical arena of our time as they do in this area. The physics of our century has taught us that there are limits to what we can measure. And in my opinion this fact alone merits strong hermeneutical interest. This is even more the case when we are concerned not just with the quantifiability of nature but with living human beings. The limits of what can be measured and, above all, of what can be effected through human intervention reach deep into the realm of health care. Health is not something that can simply be made or produced. But what then is health itself? Can it become an object for scientific investigation in the same way that it becomes an object for the individual when the balance of health is disturbed? For the ultimate aim after all must be to regain one's health and thereby to forget that one is healthy.

At the same time, the domain of science constantly extends into the realm of life itself. When it is a question of applying scientific knowledge to our own health, it is clear that we cannot be treated solely from the perspective of science. Here everyone has their own experiences and expectations. This is particularly true for all those disputed marginal areas of medical science such as pyschosomatic medicine, homoeopathy, so-called natural healing methods, hygienics, the pharmaceutical industry and all the ecological aspects involved. And this is also true for the care of the chronically ill and the old in the community. The ever growing costs involved here effectively demand that health care once again be acknowledged and recognized by the entire population as their shared responsibility.

The contributions offered here are not simply addressed to doctors, although most of them were originally presented to them as lectures, or again solely to patients, but rather to each and every one of us who must take care of our own health through the way in which we lead our lives. This particular responsibility which each person bears expands into a much broader dimension of responsibility in our highly complex civilization. Everywhere we find ourselves in possession of intensified human technical capacities which are as astounding as they are disturbing and the task is to integrate these new capacities into the social and political order as a whole. For centuries our entire culture has neglected to face up to these new demands. We have only to recall the humanitarian optimism which animated the eighteenth century and compare that with the general mood at the close of the twentieth century in this our age of mass civilization. We might think here of the immense increase in weapons technology and the destructive potential it harbours; or of the dangers posed to the conditions of human life by the technological progress from which we all benefit; and then again of the arms trade, which is as difficult to control as the drugs trade; and not least of the deluge of information which threatens to engulf our human faculty of judgement.

The enigma of health is just one small example from the range of problems which confront us. Everywhere it is a question of finding the right balance between our technical capacities and the need for responsible actions and choices. Within this whole area the problem of cultivating and caring for health represents something which directly concerns everyone. Thus we are forced to recognize that there are limits to what we can do, limits which are taught to us by illness and death. Care for our own health is an original manifestation of human existence.

Chapter 1 appeared originally in *Neue Anthropologie*, ed. Paul Vogler and H.-G. Gadamer, vol. 1 (New York and Stuttgart, 1972), pp. 9–37. It was slightly modified by the author for its first publication in English under the title 'Theory, Technology, Practice: The Task of the Science of Man', translated by Howard Brotz, in *Social Research*, vol. 44 (Fall 1977), New York. The publishers are grateful for permission to reproduce that translation here, where it appears with modifications.

Chapter 2 appeared originally in *Festschrift für Paul Vogler* (Leipzig, 1965) and was also published in vol. 1 of H.-G. Gadamer, *Kleine Schriften* (3 vols, Tübingen: J. C. B. Mohr, 1967), pp. 211–19.

Chapter 3 was given as a lecture to a meeting of the Gesamtverband Deutscher Nervenärtze in Wiesbaden in September 1963 and appeared as 'Philosophische Bemerkungen zum Problem der Intelligenz', *Der Nervenarzt*, vol. 7 (Heidelberg, 1964), pp. 281–6.

Chapter 4 was given as a radio broadcast for the Heidelberg studio of the Süddeutscher Rundfunk on 10 October 1983 and appeared in H.-G. Gadamer, *Gesammelte Werke* (Tübingen: J. C. B. Mohr, 1985–), vol. 4, pp. 288–94.

Chapter 5 appeared in *Festschrift aus Anlaß der Verleihung des Dr. Margit Egnér-Preises 1986* (Dr Margit Egnér Foundation, 1986), pp. 33–43.

Chapter 6 appeared in *Viktor von Weizsäcker zum 100. Geburtstag* (*Schriften zur anthropologischen und interdisziplinaren Forschung in der Medizin*, vol. 1), ed. Peter Hahn and Wolfgang Jacob (Berlin and Heidelberg, 1987), pp. 45–50.

Chapter 7 appeared in *Das Philosophische und die praktische Medizin* (*Brücken von der Allgemeinmedizin zur Psychosomatik*, vol. 4), ed. Helmut A. Zappe and Hansjakob Mattern (Berlin and Heidelberg, 1990), pp. 37–44.

Chapter 8 appeared in *Erfahrungsheilkunde, Acta medica empirica: Zeitschrift für ärztliche Praxis*, vol. 40, no. 11 (1991), pp. 804–8.

Chapter 9 appeared as 'Über den Zusammenhang von Autorität und kritischer Freiheit' in *Schweizer Archiv für Neurologie, Neurochirurgie und Psychiatrie*, vol. 133, no. 1 (Zurich, 1983), pp. 11–16.

Chapter 10 was given as a lecture to a conference on the work of the neurologist and psychiatrist Prince Alfred Auersperg in September 1989 in Oettingen.

Chapter 11 was given as a lecture at the University of Zurich in the summer of 1986.

Chapter 12 was given as a lecture to the Heidelberg Colloquium on the Problem of Anxiety chaired by Hermann Lang in 1990.

Chapter 13 was presented in an English translation before the Conference of Psychiatrists in San Francisco in 1989.

1

Theory, Technology, Praxis

The Change in the Meaning of Theory

'There is no doubt that all our knowledge begins with experience.' This famous beginning of Kant's *Critique of Pure Reason* surely holds too for the knowledge we possess of human beings. To begin with this includes the sum total of the ever progressing results of natural scientific research, which we call 'Science'. But then there is the empirical knowledge of so-called practice that everyone accumulates in the midst of life – the doctor, cleric, educator, judge, soldier, politician, worker, employee, official. Not only in the professional sphere but also in everyone's private and personal existence the experience that people develop out of the encounter with themselves and their fellow human beings continually grows. Beyond the domain of this experience, furthermore, there is that vast wealth of knowledge which flows towards each and every human being in the transmission of human culture – poetry, the arts as a whole, philosophy, historiography and the other historical sciences. To be sure, such knowledge is 'subjective', that is, largely unverifiable and unstable. It is, nevertheless, knowledge that science cannot ignore. As such, a rich tradition of this knowledge exists from time immemorial, from the days of Aristotle's 'practical philosophy' to the Romantic and post-Romantic age of the so-called

Geisteswissenschaften or human sciences. In contrast to the natural sciences, however, all these other sources of experience have a common quality: what we learn from them becomes experience only when actually integrated into the practical consciousness of acting human beings.

In this regard scientific experience possesses a unique status. The experience that can be validated as certain by the scientific method has the distinction of being in principle absolutely independent of any situation of action and of every integration into the context of action. This 'objectivity' conversely implies that it is able to serve every such possible context. It is precisely this 'objectivity' which was so quintessentially realized in modern science and which transformed broad expanses of the face of the earth into an artificial human environment. Now the experience which has been reworked by the sciences has, indeed, the merit of being verifiable and acquirable by everyone. But then, in addition, it raises the claim that on the basis of its methodological procedure it is the only certain experience, hence the only mode of knowing in which each and every experience is rendered truly legitimate. What we know from practical experience and the 'extra-scientific' domain must not only be subjected to scientific verification but also, should it hold its ground against this demand, belongs by this very fact to the domain of scientific research. There is in principle nothing which could not be subordinated in this manner to the competence of science.

That science not only arises from experience but according to its own methodology can be called 'experiential' or, more familiarly, 'experimental science' – an expression applicable to science only since the seventeenth century – was also articulated as a principle of modern philosophy. In the nineteenth century it led to the general conviction that people had entered into the age of 'positive' science and had left metaphysics behind. This conforms manifestly to philosophical 'positivism' in all its varieties, which rejects conceptual construction and pure speculation. But it also applies to those philosophical theories such as the Kantian which expressly point to the a priori elements in all experience. The philosophy of neo-Kantianism thus developed into a systematic theory of experience. The concept of the thing-in-itself, this 'realistic' element in the Kantian theory, was rejected by neo-Kantianism – as it was by Fichte and Hegel – as dogmatic, and reinterpreted as a concept marking the limit of the understanding. According to this theory, the object of the understanding poses an 'endless task' for definition.[1] An endless task: that is the only epistemologically tenable meaning of givenness and object. This theory has the decided merit of demonstrating the hidden dogmatism of the sensualist foundation of knowledge. The so-called givenness of perception is not given at all but presents knowledge with its task. The only 'fact' that merits this name is the fact of science.

There were, to be sure, extratheoretical spheres of validity, such as the aesthetic, which demanded recognition and thus brought forth within the neo-Kantian theory of knowledge the theme of the irrational. But that made for no change in the systematic restriction of all empirical knowledge to scientific experience. Nothing which is capable of being experienced can remain withdrawn from the competence of science. If we encounter anything unpredictable, accidental, contrary to expectations, the claim of the universality of science remains uncontestable for these things as well. What seems to be something irrational is, in the eyes of the scientist, a phenomenon on the frontier of science; this is how phenomena appear on that border where science finds applications to practice. What occurs in practice as the unexpected and mostly undesirable consequences of the application of science is seen as something altogether different from the irreducible irrationality of chance. According to the essential character of science, this presents nothing more than a task for further research. The progress of science is sustained by its continual self-correction. And practice which is based on the application of science likewise requires that science further and further improve, by continual self-correction, the reliability of the expectations placed upon it.

But what does practice in the above sense mean? Is the application of science as such practice? Is all practice the application of science? Even if the application of science enters into all practice, the two are still not identical. For practice means not only the making of whatever one can make; it is also choice and decision between possibilities. Practice always has a relationship to a person's 'being'. This is reflected in the figurative expression, *Was machst Du denn?*, which does not ask, literally, what are you *doing* but, rather, how *are* you? From this point of view an irreducible opposition between science and practice becomes evident. Science is essentially incomplete; whereas practice requires instant decisions. The incompleteness of all experimental science thus means that it not only raises a legitimate claim of universality, by virtue of its readiness to process new experience, but also is not wholly able to make good this claim. Practice requires knowledge, which means that it is obliged to treat the knowledge available at the time as complete and certain. The knowledge known from science, however, is not of this sort. There is thus a fundamental difference between modern science and the premodern aggregate of knowledge, which under the name 'philosophy' comprehended all human knowledge. This difference is precisely that what we know from 'science' is incomplete and, therefore, can no longer be called a 'doctrine'. It consists of nothing other than the current state of 'research'.

One must make clear the full significance of the innovation which came into the world with the experimental sciences and their underlying idea of method. If one contrasts 'science' with the whole of that knowledge of former times derived from the heritage of antiquity and which was still dominant throughout the high Middle Ages, it is apparent that the conceptions both of theory and of practice have fundamentally changed. Naturally there was always application of knowledge to practice, as indicated by the very terms 'sciences' and 'arts' (*epistemai* and *technai*). 'Science' was after all but the highest intensification of the knowledge that guided practice. It understood itself, however, as pure *theoria*, that is, as knowledge sought for its own sake and not for its practical significance. It was in the Greek idea of science that the relation between theory in this precise sense and practice first came to a critical point as a problem. While the mathematical knowledge of the Egyptian geometricians or the Babylonian astronomers was nothing other than a store of knowledge that had accumulated out of practice and for practice, the Greeks transformed this know-how and knowledge into a knowledge of principles and thus into demonstrable knowledge which one became aware of to enjoy for its own sake out of, so to speak, a primary curiosity about the world. Out of this spirit arose Greek science and mathematics, as well as the enlightenment of Greek natural philosophy and, despite its essential relation to practice, Greek medicine as well. Here for the first time science and its application, theory and practice, parted ways.

Yet this divergence can hardly be compared to the modern relation between theory and practice, which was formed by the seventeenth-century idea of science. For science is no longer the totality of the knowledge of the world and of humankind, which Greek philosophy, whether as philosophy of nature or as practical philosophy, had elaborated and articulated in the communicative form of language. The foundation of modern science is experience in a wholly new sense. With the idea of the unitary method of the understanding, as formulated by Descartes in his *Rules*, the ideal of certainty became the standard for all understanding. Only that which could be verified could have validity as experience. In the seventeenth century, experience thus ceased to be a source or starting point of knowledge but became, in the sense of 'experiment', a tribunal of verification before which the validity of mathematically projected laws could be confirmed or refuted. Galileo did not happen to acquire the laws of free-falling objects from experience but, as he himself says, they came from conceptual projection: 'mente concipio,' that is, 'I conceive' – or, more precisely, 'I project in my mind.' What Galileo thus 'projected' in the idea of a free-falling object was certainly no object of experience: a vacuum does not exist in nature. What he understood, however, precisely by this abstraction were laws within the skein of causal relationships, which are intertwined and cannot be disentangled in concrete experience. The mind isolates the individual relationships and by measuring and weighing determines the exact contribution of each; it thereby opens up the possibility of intentionally bringing out factors of a causal kind. It is thus not altogether wrong to say that modern natural science – without detracting from the purely theoretical interest that animates it – means not so much knowledge as know-how. This means that it is practice.[2] It would appear to me more correct, however, to say that science makes possible knowledge directed to the power of making, a knowing mastery of nature. This is technology. And this is precisely what practice is not. For the former is not knowledge which, as steadily increasing experience, is acquired from practice, the life situation, and the circumstances of action. On the contrary, it is a kind of knowledge which for the first time makes possible a novel relation to practice, namely, that of constructive projection and application. It is of the essence of its procedure to achieve in all spheres the abstraction which isolates individual causal relationships. This is the unavoidable particularity of its competence which it has to accept as part of the bargain. What in fact emerged, however, was 'science', with its new notion of theory as well as practice. This is a true event in the history of humankind, which conferred a new social and political accent on science.

The Impact of Technology on Modern Man

It is thus not for nothing that one calls our present age an age of the sciences. There are above all two grounds on which to justify this assertion. First, the scientific-technical mastery of nature has at this moment acquired proportions which qualitatively differentiate our century from earlier centuries. Science, obviously, has become today the primary productive factor of the human economy. But beyond this its practical application has created what is in principle a new situation. No longer is it limited to the premodern implications of *techne*, namely, to filling out the possibilities of further development left open by nature (Aristotle). It has moved upward to the level of an artificial counterpart to reality. Formerly, the modification of our environment was due more or less to natural causes, for example, change in climate (the Ice Age), the influence of the weather (erosion, sedimentation, etc.), droughts, formation of swamps and the like. Only occasionally was it due to the intervention of human beings. Such interventions were perhaps the deforestation of woods, which turned into barren lands as a consequence, the extinction of animal species through hunting, the exhaustion of soils through cultivation, the drying up of the resources in the ground as the result of exploitation. These were always more or less irreversible modifications. In such cases, however, mankind either saved itself by finding new places to live or learned to prevent the consequences in due time. As for the rest, the contribution of human labour, of the gatherer, the hunter, or the farmer, brought about no real disturbance to the equilibrium of nature.

Today, however, the technical exploitation of natural resources and the artificial transformation of our environment has become so carefully planned and extensive that its consequences endanger the natural cycle of things and bring about irreversible developments on a large scale. The problem of the protection of the environment is the visible expression of this totalization of technical civilization. Obviously, more significant tasks fall upon the shoulders of science, and it must plead in their behalf before that public consciousness which the effects of our technical civilization are beginning to reach. On the one hand this leads to the emotional blindness with which a mass critique of culture reacts to these phenomena, and it is necessary to avert in time the iconoclasm which threatens from this quarter. On the other hand there is the superstitious faith in science which strengthens the technocratic unscrupulousness with which technical know-how spreads without restraint. In both respects science must carry on a kind of demythologization of itself and indeed by its very own means: critical information and methodical discipline. Issues such as the city, the environment, population growth, the world food supply, problems of the aged, etc., thus justly acquire a privileged place among the scientific themes of our knowledge of man. The atom bomb proves itself more and more to be only a special case of the self-endangering of human beings and their life on this planet to which science has led, and which it has to do its utmost to avert.

Within science itself, however, there is also the threat of a similar danger of self-destruction which arises directly out of the perfection of the modern business of research. The specialization of research has long since moved away from that orientation towards the whole which as late as the eighteenth century still made possible an encyclopedic knowledge. Even in the beginning of our own century there were still enough paths of well-organized information which made it widely possible for the layperson to partake of scientific knowledge and for the researcher to partake in other sciences. Since then, however, the worldwide expansion of research and its increasing specialization have led to a deluge of information which turns against itself. Professional librarians today carefully consider how they should store and administer – and administration means here expansion – the masses of information which increase alarmingly year in and year out. Specialized researchers find themselves in need of an orientation which is similar to that of the layperson in general as soon as they look beyond the most limited range of their area of work. And this is often necessary for the researchers who find themselves no longer able to do justice to the new problems which they take up with the older methods of their own science. It remains altogether necessary for laypeople who for their political action want not only to be guided by prepared information but to form a judgement. In this flood of information the orientation of the layperson is peculiarly mediated and, hence, dependent.

With this we come to the second sphere in which science has become a new kind of factor in human life, and this is its application to the life of society itself. Today the social sciences aspire towards fundamentally altering the practice of human living together that was shaped by traditions and institutions. Science raises the claim – and it does this on the basis of the technical state of civilization today – of putting social life as well on rational foundations and of freeing the unquestionable authority of tradition from taboo. This occurs explicitly in the case of ideological criticism when it seeks to transform social consciousness by emancipatory reflection, seeing repressive compulsions at work in the structure of economic and social authority. More effective yet, however, because it touches each and every one, is the silent form in which more and more areas of human life are subjected to technical domination, where rational automata take the place of the personal decision of individuals and groups.

This represents a fundamental alteration in our life. It is the more remarkable in so far as it is a question less of scientific-technical progress as such than of resolute rationality in the application of science, which overcomes with a new uninhibitedness the durability of custom as well as the restraints present within a 'world view'. Formerly the consequences opened up for us by the new possibilities of scientific progress remained limited at every step by the norms which prevailed, unquestioned and self-evident, in our cultural and religious tradition. One may perhaps recall what emotions were unleashed in the past by the struggle over Darwinism. It took decades until dispassionate, objective discussion became possible; and even today Darwinism still moves people's passions. The natural scientific knowledge of Darwin is, of course, today uncontested; but its application to social life remains exposed to manifold objections. Without taking a stand about the question in this case, one may establish as a principle that the application of scientific understanding to areas where what is called today the self-understanding of man is at stake not only often leads to conflict but also necessarily invokes extra-scientific considerations which defend a right of their own.

Thus today one sees science itself in conflict with our human consciousness of value. I am thinking here of the horrifying perspectives which have been developed on the basis of modern genetics pointing to the alteration of heredity and planned breeding. That does not, indeed, have the dramatic power to shock that Darwinism formerly had. It also does not have the horrible obviousness such as that which the use of atomic energy had for the destruction of human life in Hiroshima. But in the consciousness of all researchers the warning has been emerging that they possess a heightened responsibility for the future of mankind.

When we ask ourselves how this general state of our consciousness is reflected in the main positions assumed by present-day students in anthropology and philosophy, the answer is very varied. A certain more or less well-known standpoint still remains the critique of the traditional assertion of the special place of humankind in the cosmos, which in the face of the progress of the natural scientific understanding unmasks itself more and more as a residual prejudice of theology. It enters into the themes of our knowledge of man, wherever the characterization of human beings relative to animals is at issue. This may be precisely the reason why research into behavior today is now enjoying an unaccustomed resurgence of publicity, formerly in the work of Uexküll, today in that of Lorenz and his pupils.[3]

No one today can imagine that we are really able to perfect the integration we require for our knowledge of humankind. Our progress of knowledge is subject to the law of increasing specialization and, hence, to increasing obstacles to comprehensiveness. The action of human beings – that is, the conscious use of human knowledge and know-how for the preservation of health or social equilibrium, particularly peace – manifestly lacks a unified scientific basis. It is inevitable that it seeks at times to create this for itself by means of assumptions about a world-view. In retrospect we easily perceive what takes place quite unperceived in the present, namely, how certain insights acquire the power of fascination and then become magnified into a general frame of reference. Such, for example, is the superstructure of the science of mechanics and its transfer to other areas, with all its further developments – with others still to come – produced by cybernetics. Similar in its dogmatic character is the prevalence of the concepts of consciousness and will. The concepts of consciousness, self-consciousness and will, in the form to which they were led by philosophical Idealism, dominated both the theory of knowledge in the nineteenth century and its psychology. This is an outstanding example of the significance which theoretical concepts can possess for applications to the study of man.

This is not the place to analyse the dogmatism in the concept of consciousness as well as in the concept of the soul, a dogmatism which lies in the concept of representation or the content of consciousness on the one hand, and in the concept of the faculties of the soul on the other. It suffices to note the fate of the principle of self-consciousness. This principle, in Kant's concept of the transcendental synthesis of apperception, lay at the basis of the Idealistic position. It radiated back as far as Descartes, and forward to Husserl. It succumbed to a critique which began with Nietzsche and became victorious in various ways in our century – for example, through Freud or Heidegger.

For present purposes this critique means, among other things, that the social role of individuals rather than their self-understanding moves into the foreground. What does the self-maintaining identity of the ego mean? Does the ego that vouches for itself in self-consciousness even exist? What is the source of the continuity of its self-sameness? One answer is the 'struggle for recognition', which Hegel described as the dialectic of self-consciousness. Or – antithetically – there is the Christian inwardness for which Kierkegaard, in the sense of 'choice', laid the basis with the ethical concept of continuity. Or is the ego but a subsidiary creation of unity between alternate roles? One thinks here of how Brecht, in *The Good Person of Szechuan* as well as in his theory of the epic theatre, disputes the legitimacy of the old dramaturgical idea of the unity of character. The direction of behaviourist research also presents an example of this dedogmatizing of self-consciousness. The abandonment of the 'internality of the psychical', which is the basis of it, is a positive indication that behaviour patterns are now being studied which are common to animals and humans and which are wholly inaccessible via such a concept as self-understanding.[4]

Yet the contribution of philosophical anthropology to the science of humankind remains considerable, even after the theology of the soul and the mythology of self-consciousness have succumbed to criticism. When seen within the totality of the research situation, the contribution of philosophical anthropology over against the scientific models which cybernetics and physics have to offer would still appear to be of greater heuristic fruitfulness. Indeed, modern theoretical and physiological research on the relationship of consciousness and body or soul and body shows an impressive methodical caution and a gift of invention. Likewise it is impressive to learn from biology and behavioural research how continuous are the transitions from animal to human behaviour and that one cannot so easily explain, purely from the standpoint of behaviour, the 'leap' to humanity by the specific peculiarities which distinguish humans from the other animals. The progress of research shows that the anti-evolutionary passion which burst forth in the struggle over Darwinism plays no further role today. But precisely when one pushes the human as near to the animal as the phenomena permit and require – and with regard to modes of behaviour, that is astonishingly far – the unique position of human beings surprisingly reveals itself in a particularly vivid fashion. Precisely in their full naturalness they appear as something extraordinary; and the evident fact that no other living being makes its own environment into a cultural world as does man, who became thereby 'Lord of Creation', has within it a new unbiblical power of revelation. It teaches no longer that the soul is of an otherworldly order but, on the contrary, that nature does not have the meaning which the investigation of nature of the past centuries required us to think it had, namely, as 'matter subject to laws' (Kant). The 'frugality of nature', which was a fruitful teleological key conception in the age of mechanics and even today still finds manifold confirmation, is not the only point of view from which to think about nature. For the evolution of life is just as much an event of enormous prodigality.

The standpoints both of self-preservation and of adaptation are losing their key function in research into living beings. The philosophy of institutions, in which Gehlen interpreted the latter as compensation for the biological deficiency of endowment of the 'as yet undefined animal', which according to Nietzsche is what man is, is also affected by this new tendency.[5] Studies of biologists, ethnologists, historians and philosophers are in agreement that humans are not humans because they dispose of an additional endowment which relates them to an otherworldly order (Scheler's concept of spirit).[6] But they also all hold that the point of view of inherent deficiencies does not suffice to explain their distinctiveness. On the contrary, what is apparent is the profusion of human capacities and abilities for perception and movement, the unequal distribution of which is characteristic. Plessner called this the 'eccentricity', of human beings.[7] It distinguishes them in that they expresses themselves in behaviour by means of the body – for example, in gestures – but also can, by willing and acting, go beyond the natural endowment of a living being. This is seen, for example, in their behaviour to other human beings and in particular through the 'invention' of war. In this regard, modern psychology also is once again taking a significant stand, precisely because it combines the methods of research of the natural and social sciences with the hermeneutical sciences and tests out the most different methods on the same object.

It is by virtue of the 'eccentric' constitution of human life that the differentiated modes originate in which human eccentricity is worked out. We call this humanity's culture. Not only do the great themes of economy, law, language, religion, science and philosophy bear witness to it as the objective traces which humanity has left behind; there is also, as its other source, the knowledge of themselves which human beings acquire and transmit. Plessner comprehends all this in the formulation that man 'embodies himself'.[8] Here arises and flows forth that other source of knowledge of humankind which is prior to natural science and which has given and shaped as a theme for researchers into nature their manifold contributions to the knowledge of humankind. For thanks to the knowledge humans have of themselves, the 'science' which seeks to perceive everything that becomes accessible to it with its methodical means is confronted in a special way with the theme 'human being'. Its task of understanding is posed to it as one that is unending, incomplete, continually in view.

What is this knowledge which human beings possess of themselves? Is it possible to understand 'self-consciousness' with the means of science? Does it represent a theoretical objectification of a person which may be compared to the mode of the objectification possessed by an artifact or a tool, which can be designed in advance from a blueprint? Manifestly not. It is true that human consciousness itself, in addition, can in a complicated way be made the object of natural-scientific research. Information theory and machine technology can become fruitful for research about human beings since they clarify the functional mode of human consciousness through their models. But this model construction does not claim to *control* scientifically the organic and conscious life of a person. It is satisfied to elucidate by means of simulation the highly complicated mechanism which permits living reactions and particularly human consciousness to function. Now one may ask whether this is not simply an expression of the fact that cybernetics is still stuck wholly at its beginnings and therefore is not yet adequate to its own goal, namely, the natural-scientific understanding of such highly complicated systems. It seems reasonable to me, however, to imagine for a moment a perfected cybernetics for which the difference between machine and living person had really disappeared. Our knowledge about humanity would then find its perfection in its ability to make such machines. With regard to this point one must take to heart Steinbuch's warning that fundamentally there are 'no insights of automation theory or language theory which make possible any differentiation between what man can do and what automatons *cannot* do'.

We are not concerned here, however, with the know-how of machines or the know-how of those who use them. The question is rather what human beings, with their know-how, want. 'Can' a machine also want? That would also mean, can it 'not want' to do something it 'can' do? In other words, is the perfected automaton the ideal of a useful human being? Throughout much of the labour process it is in fact an ideal substitute for the power of human labour; and one of the greatest problems of the future – comparable to what occurred after the introduction of mechanical looms – may become that of integrating these machines into economic and social life.

To this degree automation touches social practice – but, so to speak, from outside. It does not lessen the distance between human being and machine but makes its irreducibility visible. Even the most useful human beings for the one who makes use of them are still fellow human beings and have knowledge of themselves. This is not only a self-consciousness of know-how, such as the ideal self-regulating machine might possess, but is, rather, a social consciousness which governs the one who uses another just as much as it does the latter, or, to put it differently, governs all who have their place within the social process of labour. Even the mere usufructuary has such a place, if only indirectly.

Thus, from the end-point of a perfected technology, what was from the very first the proper human meaning of 'practice' becomes clear. It is characterized by that very possibility of human behaviour which we call 'theoretical'. This belongs to the fundamental constitution of human 'practice'. Because of this, human know-how and knowledge is perennially not only that which is acquired by learning and experience; it is also the autonomization of means into tools which raises to a higher power the human capacity to learn and to bequeath human know-how to future generations. Implicit in this is intelligent control of the causal context which enables us to direct in a planned way our own behaviour. But this also demands conscious ordering into a system of ends. It will be found that the other main statement of modern research – namely, that human language is fundamentally distinguished from the sign systems of animal communication – also conforms to the oldest insights of Greek thought. This is so in so far as language enables us to make facts and their contexts objective – and this means, of course, to make them openly available in advance for any possible form of human behaviour. The use of means for different ends and the use of different means for the same end depend on this, as does the order of preference among the ends themselves.

The ability to behave theoretically thus is in itself part of the practice of humankind. It is clear without further ado that it was the 'theoretical' gift of humanity which made it possible for human beings to establish distance from the immediate aims of their desires, to restrain their desires, as Hegel put it, and with this to lay the basis of an 'objective behaviour', which manifests itself in the production of tools as well as in human speech. From this arises as a further basis of distanciation the possibility of socially ordering, by the ends of the society, all that we do or fail to do.

Obviously, there is a problem of integration in the simplest relationship between knowing and doing. At least since the advent of the division of labour, human knowledge has developed in such a way that it has the quality of specialization which must be expressly learned. There is then this problem for practice: knowledge, which can be transmitted independently of the situation of action and can thus be detached from the practical context of action, needs to be applied at times in a new situation of human action. Now the general empirical knowledge of human beings which decisively affects their practical decisions is inseparable from the knowledge which has been transmitted by specialized knowledge. What is more, it is an absolute moral duty to pursue knowledge to the greatest possible degree; that means today that one must also be informed by means of 'science'. Max Weber's famous distinction between the ethics of pure intention and the ethics of responsibility was decided in favour of the latter in the moment it was laid down.[9] Thus the entire abundance of information which modern science can produce from its partial vantage points about the human can never be excluded from the orbit of what is practically of interest for humankind. Nevertheless, in this lies the problem. All practical decisions of human beings depend indeed on their general knowledge. Yet a specific difficulty lies in applying this knowledge in the concrete case. It is the task of the power of judgement (and not, to repeat, of teaching and learning) to recognize in a given situation the applicability of a general rule. This task exists wherever knowledge in general is to be applied; the problem is irreducible. There are, however, spheres of practical behaviour in which this difficulty does not culminate in a critical conflict. That is true for the whole sphere of technical experience, that is, of making. There practical empirical knowledge is built up step by step as it is moulded by the encounter with experience. The general knowledge which science acquires, since it grasps the bases of the events, can take its place alongside this empirical knowledge, and can also serve it as a corrective, but does not render it dispensable.

However, even in this simplest case of knowledge directed towards production, the very idea of which shows the two-sidedness of knowledge and know-how, tensions can emerge; and under the conditions of the modern business of science this simple relation between 'theoretical knowledge' and practical action is increasingly attenuated. Moreover, the term 'business of science' has already become a catchword which points to the qualitative difference between knowledge and action present within the extreme attenuation of their relationship.

The institutionalization of science into a business belongs to the larger context of economic and social life in the industrial age. Not only is science a business, but all the work performed in modern life is organized like a business. The individual, with a definite assignment of work to do, is fitted into a larger business-like whole, which on its part within the highly specialized organization of modern work has a function which is strictly provided for. But this means at the same time that the function is one which is discharged without its own orientation to the whole. While the virtues of accommodation and adjustment to such rational forms of organization are correspondingly cultivated, the autonomy of the formation of judgement and of action according to one's own judgement are correspondingly neglected. That has its basis in the character of modern civilization and permits the following to be pronounced as a general rule: the more rationally the organizational forms of life are shaped, the less is rational judgement exercised and trained among individuals. Modern traffic psychology, to illustrate this by an example, knows the dangers which lie in the automation of the regulation of traffic. Drivers find fewer and fewer opportunities for an autonomously free decision in their behaviour and thus more and more unlearn how to make such decisions rationally.

The tension between theoretical knowledge and practical application that is inherent in the modern condition can be continually bridged to the extent that science also deals thematically with the problem of application of its respective subject-matter and as applied science concerns itself with this problem. The entire content of what we call technology has this character of being applied science. As such, however, the tension in no way disappears but in fact only increases, as the rule stated above also asserts. One can at this point also express it as follows: the more strongly the sphere of application becomes rationalized, the more does proper exercise of judgement along with practical experience in the proper sense of the term fail to take place.

This is a process of a two-sided sort, for it also involves the relation between producer and consumer. The spontaneity of the user of technology is in fact more and more eliminated precisely by this technology. Users must accommodate themselves to the rules of its ends and to that extent renounce their 'freedom'. They become dependent on the correct functioning of the technology.

But then there arises for people in this kind of dependence a yet wholly different lack of freedom. There is the artificial creation of needs, above all by means of modern advertising. In principle what is at stake is dependence on the means of information. The consequence of this condition is that both the specialist who acquires new information and the journalist – that is, the informed informer – become social factors in their own right. The journalist is well informed and decides how far others should be informed. The specialist presents us with an unassailable judgement. If no one other than the specialist is able to judge the specialist, and if even misadventures or mistakes can be criticized only by specialists – one thinks of the 'malpractice' of doctors or architects – an area thereby has become in a precise sense autonomous. The appeal to science is irrefutable.

The Primacy of Practice

The unavoidable consequence is that science is invoked far beyond the limits of its real competence. This includes, not least of all, the self-evident range of its own application. It is the merit of the American sociologist Freidson to have looked closely at the 'autonomization' that is expanding, by virtue of the appeal to science, in the practical professions, particularly in the medical profession.[10] He has correctly given the prominence it deserves to the point that pure medical science as such is not competent for the practical application of its knowledge because all sorts of other considerations, evaluations, customary practices, preferences, and even personal interests enter into the picture. From the standpoint of science, which the author assumes with the full rigour of 'critical rationality', the appeal to 'wisdom' is not even valid.

Freidson sees in this appeal nothing but the authoritarian mask of the experts who protect themselves from the objections of the layperson. To raise a standard of objective science to such an extreme is indeed a very one-sided perspective. The criticism, however, of the social and political claims of the experts can in the case of such an appeal to 'wisdom' be quite healthy. It defends the ideal of the free society. By virtue of such criticism citizens make the claim that they will not be disenfranchised by the authority of the experts. All this has a special relevance to the sphere of medical science and art. In the very way in which we describe the discipline we vacillate between the terms science and art, and the insight given by the history of medicine into the tension that marks their relationship is striking. This is linked to the special quality of the art of healing, namely, that this art, unlike the arts for producing artifacts, has as its task the restoration of something natural. Precisely because medicine is concerned with techniques for making artifacts within only a limited extent (since ancient times in dentistry and astonishingly early also in surgery), there still exists, even today, a particularly wide scope for the exercise of the doctor's power of judgement. Everything which we call diagnosis is indeed in formal respects the subsumption of a given case under the generalities of an illness. But in this very 'knowing how to distinguish', which is the real meaning of diagnosis, lies the true art. Certainly both general and specialized medical knowledge belong to this art. But they are not sufficient for it. Misdiagnoses, cases of false subsumption under a universal principle, are in general to be charged not, obviously, to the science but to the art and ultimately to the judgement of the doctor.

Now the craft of doctors is distinguished by the fact that they not only must maintain or restore a natural equilibrium, as is also the case in agriculture or in the breeding of animals, but also are involved with human beings who must be 'treated'. This again limits the range of the scientific competence of doctors. As such, their knowledge is in principle different from that of the craftsman. The craftsman's art can easily defend its competence against the objections of the layperson. The craftsman's knowledge or know-how finds its confirmation in the success of what it does. The craftsman, moreover, acts by order, and in the final analysis it is use which lays down the standards to be followed. In so far as the order is clear, the craftsman possesses unlimited and uncontested competence. That is rarely the case with an architect or a tailor, because the people who give the order seldom really know what they want. In principle, however, the giving of an order to a craftsman as well as its acceptance is something that is a binding contract, binding together both of the parties with their respective obligations, whose claims are proven by the unambiguous character of a produced piece of work.

In contrast, there is for the doctor no such demonstrable 'work'. The health of the patient cannot be regarded in this way. Although health is naturally the goal of the doctor's activity, it is not actually 'made' by the doctor. Connected to this is something further: the goal of health is not a condition that is clearly definable from within the medical art. For illness is a social state of affairs. It is also a psychological-moral state of affairs, much more than a fact that is determinable from within the natural sciences. All this, which formerly made the family doctor a friend of the family, indicates the elements of medical efficacy of which we today are often painfully deprived. But even today the doctor's power of persuasion as well as the trust and the cooperation of the patient constitute essential therapeutic factors which belong to a wholly different dimension than that of the physical-chemical influences of medications upon the organism or of 'medical intervention'.

The example of the doctor thus shows with special clarity how the relationship between theory and practice comes to a critical point under the conditions of modern science. There is first of all the diagnosis. Today this calls into play such a specialized technology that for the most part there hardly remains anything for the doctor to do but to expose the patient to the anonymity of the clinical apparatus. Very often this is also the case with the treatment. This has its consequences for the whole. In contrast to the family doctors of the old school, the practical experience of clinicians, who in general see their patients only in the clinical stage, is unavoidably abstract. The inverse, however, also applies to general practitioners today. Even if they still make house calls, they on their part can get only a reduced opportunity for experience. The example thus teaches us that while the development of practical technologies, to judge from appearances, reduces the distance between the general knowledge of the science and the correct decisions of the moment, the qualitative difference between practical knowledge and scientific knowledge actually increases. Precisely because the technologies which are applied are indispensable, the sphere of judgement and experience, out of which the right practical decisions are made, gets smaller. What modern medicine can do is astonishing. But in spite of all the progress which the natural sciences have brought about for our knowledge of sickness and health, and in spite of the enormous expenditure on rationalized technology for diagnosis and treatment which has taken place in this area, the sphere of the unrationalized element within it is particularly high. This shows itself in the fact that even now, as in the oldest times, the idea of the good doctor or even of the medical genius has much more of the prized esteem we think characteristic of an artist than of a man of science. Thus in this case one may less than elsewhere deny the irreplaceability of practical experience and the impossibility of circumventing it. The appeal to 'wisdom', the claim to be a 'wise' doctor, may be an illegitimate means of compulsion where it is raised – that is what it amounts to in the end wherever one appeals to one's 'authority'. As it is a sign, however, of an intensified state of delusion to regard authority simply as something illegitimate which one would be better off replacing by 'rational' forms of decision-making – as if one could eliminate the weight of true authority in any form of human social organization – so too the share which 'experience' has in making one prudent, thinking precisely but not only of the doctor here, is just as undemonstrable as it is convincing.

One will find in all spheres of practical application of rules, and thus in what one calls in general 'practice', that the more one 'masters' one's know-how the more one possesses freedom vis-à-vis this know-how. Those who 'master' their art need to prove their superiority neither to themselves nor to others. It is old Platonic wisdom that true know-how makes possible precisely a certain distanciation from it. It is thus the master runner who can also run 'slowly' the best, the one who really knows who can also lie most effectively, etc. What Plato is saying here implicitly is that it is this freedom vis-à-vis one's own know-how which in fact liberates for the perspective of authentic practice what transcends the competence of the know-how – what Plato calls 'the good', which determines our practical-political decisions.

Precisely in the context of the medical art, we speak of yet another mode of 'mastery'. The doctor masters not only his or her art (as does every capable person); we also say of medical science that it 'masters' or learns to master certain diseases. In this expression the special character of medical know-how is articulated, namely, that it does not 'make' and 'produce' but cooperates in the recovery of the ill. To 'master' a disease thus means to know its course and to be able to control it – not to be master of 'nature' to such a degree that one could simply 'take away' the disease. In the place where medicine most closely approximates to a technical art, namely, surgery, we also speak in this way. But even surgeons know that 'intervention remains intervention.' Thus they, too, when making their decision, will always have to look beyond what their medical competence encompasses. And the more certainly they 'master' their art, the more free they will be in confronting it, and not simply in the sphere of medical 'practice' itself.

The Task of a Comprehensive Science of Humankind

The tension between the specialized knowledge of today and the conditions of practice is thus extremely large. The clarification of the interdisciplinary methodological context within which individual researchers move will only occasionally be productive for them. Moreover, let it not be denied that one of the unavoidable consequences of the modern organization of research is that the horizon of the specialist becomes focused on the methodological and intellectual state of the specialty. The comprehensive task consists of bringing out the true character of careful and provisional research, in the face of the expectations and speculations of the layperson – and in neighbouring areas the researcher is also a layperson. It is a corrective of a special kind to be aware of the disputability – that is, the provisional and in each case limited character – of that which science knows. Science is thus able to combat the superstition that it can relieve individuals of responsibility for their own practical decisions.

We may ask: does not modern science really investigate more and more spheres and thereby make them subject to scientific control? And surely it is true that in whatever area science knows something the layperson's knowledge loses its practical legitimacy. Nevertheless it remains true that each person's practical action continually crosses the boundary of this sphere. This applies, as we have seen, even to specialists themselves when they must act practically on the basis of their own competence. The practical consequences of their knowledge are not simply subordinate to their own intellectual competence itself. This is all the more true of the great domain of human decisions regarding family, society and state, for which the specialist does not have sufficient practically relevant knowledge to offer and which everyone must decide 'according to their own best knowledge and conscience'.

Thus we ask once again: what can a science of humankind that faces this fact achieve for humanity's knowledge of itself? What can it practically bring about? The fashionable answer today to such questions speaks about a 'change of consciousness'. In fact, one can conceive of this taking place with the doctor, the teacher, and perhaps every other specialist, where they become mindful of the limits of their specializations. They then become ready to acknowledge experiences which are uncomfortable for the private interests of researchers – such as, for example, the social and political responsibility present in every profession where others are dependent upon someone. Since the horrors of atomic warfare penetrated the general consciousness, the term 'responsibility of science' has acquired great popularity. That the specialist is not only a specialist but also a socially and politically responsible agent, is however, fundamentally nothing new. The Platonic Socrates met his ruin for laying bare the inability of the specialist to rise to this level of responsibility. The moral-philosophical reflection of antiquity thus already posed for itself the question of how far such responsibility extends in view of the unpredictability of the use and abuse of the products of human handiwork. It sought its answer in the domain of 'practical philosophy' by subjecting all the 'arts' to 'political' ordering. Today there is a need of this on a worldwide scale, given the inexorable transformation of all scientific know-how into technology, within the existing economic order, as soon as something promises a profit.

One can also describe the change by saying that a corresponding development of a social-political consciousness has not kept pace with the scientific enlightenment and the technical progress of our civilization. Moreover, the immensely increased possibilities of application which science has created for the shaping of society may be only in the beginning stage. One must thus say that the progress of technology encounters an unprepared humanity. It vacillates between the extremes of an affect-laden opposition to rational innovation and a no less affect-laden craving to 'rationalize' all forms and sectors of life, a development which more and more acquires the form of a panic flight from freedom. Thus the question becomes more acute of how far science itself should assume a shared responsibility for the consequences of its forms of technical application. Moreover the fact remains that the immanent and consistent structure of research has a necessary character of its own. Herein lies the non-negotiable right to the demand for freedom of research. Research manifestly can flourish only at the risk of conjuring up the fateful experience of the sorcerer's apprentice. Every addition to knowledge is, regarding its significance and consequences, unpredictable.

Thus we are not going to be able to speak seriously about charging science as such with the responsibility for the consequences of its progress. This would automatically have the most undesired effects: the dread of responsibility, preference for the 'safe' paths of research, bureaucratization, superficial labelling, and finally aimless drifting. Yet it is true that science acquires an influence on our life to an increasing degree and, therefore, that the consequences of research possess an ever greater human significance. One thinks simply of the development of chemical fertilization, of chemical preservatives, of the problem of waste disposal (not only in the production of atomic energy but above all in the use of synthetic materials), of water and air pollution. How far must science accept the responsibility for this?

Here too science can only be responsible for what it alone has always been responsible for – that is, in all these matters, to recognize and to seize tasks for inquiry, thereby serving the scientific and practical mastery of the problems which it and its application have created. One therefore asks whether there should not be metasciences – futurology, the science of planning, etc – expressly to take up this task. But in every case this only displaces still further the locus of the ultimate decisions. In other words, it is the task not of science but of politics to supervise the application of the know-how made possible by science. It is also conversely the task not of politics but of science to supervise its own needs, investments in time and money, etc. This is in the final analysis the function of scientific criticism.

But here too the relation between theory and practice is extremely complicated. The theoretical interest (and the prerequisites in life for 'leisure') do not suffice where the business of science itself has become an organized whole, with a division of labour and a large budget. Research needs the political sphere to an extreme degree. Inversely, the political human being – and everyone is such who has a share in political decisions through action or inaction – is more and more dependent on scientific information. This places an increased responsibility on researchers in view of the increased significance which the results of their research can have. They must make its necessity convincing. To this end they must appeal to the general faculty of judgement. They themselves, however, must possess such a faculty of judgement in order to control their own egoism as specialists. It seems to me that here the science of humankind has a further task. The voice of all researchers who look back on their life's work and reflect on its anthropological significance can expect a heightened interest among all whose social and political consciousness requires information from science. The general question, of what one can say today about problems of human practice from the standpoint of science, becomes linked to the other question: what practical-political consequences do leading researchers draw from their scientific knowledge? With regard to the latter question one must keep clearly in mind that the perspectives of competent researchers are indeed distinguished by their level of information. But as practical and political perspectives they cannot claim the same competence and authority which belongs to the body of information as such. The latter is only a contributing element to the practical deliberation and decision that everyone, by virtue of their own responsibility, performs.

In all this nothing has been said about the credulous separation between information and a practical or political grasp of things. Yet the concept of information, as developed by cybernetics, creates a problem of its own as soon as it involves the practical knowledge of man. What faces us is an 'anthropological' problem. We know it as the practical task of getting correct information. Naturally every machine which stores information carries out certain choices which originate in the programming. It is thus able to take the information which flows into it and continually separate it out again. But it forgets nothing. An enormous superiority, we may perhaps think, which will cause us constantly to complain about the limits of the human memory. But the machine, which forgets nothing, cannot as such remember. Forgetting is not exactly separating out, but it is not simply storing. It is a kind of latency which maintains its own presence. Everything hinges on the character of this presence. To be sure, stored information which one can call forth from a machine has a kind of latent presence. But precisely herein lies the difference. The machine can well exhibit the neurophysiological state called *mneme*. It can also – perhaps some day – imitate the neurophysiological process of 'recollection' (seeking and finding) or that of 'passive' recollection by means of 'a sudden flash of thought'. To this extent it 'explains' forgetting and remembering. But it does not 'know how' to do it by itself, precisely because forgetting is not a 'knowing how'.

What is involved in this may become clear to the layperson by the example of a word index. The pride of a mechanized index is its completeness. It is guaranteed to forget or omit nothing. Naturally one quickly realizes that such completeness also has its practical disadvantages. A word that appears frequently fills many pages of the index. This at once creates its own form of hiding place for what one is seeking. One then tells oneself that a sought-for word becomes recognizable only through its context. The context index is thus the next step towards making a mechanized index practically useful. But here too the idea of the context is feasible only in an abstractly isolating form. The actual context within which the actual user is really seeking something is not capable, moreover, of classification. Granted, such an index is objective and attains the full objectivity of the given text. Granted, every selective index signifies a subjective interpretation of the text. Granted, this is deplored by every individual user as a defect. For that reason the users will find useful not the 'perfected' index but only the index which corresponds with their own subjective points of view. And that is the one which they compile themselves. Only such an index is so selected that it potentially 'reminds' in all its data. It 'reminds' as the presentation given by the context index of the machine is unable to do. This is so because the latter does not rediscover in itself individual memory traces but necessarily offers everything that it 'knows'. Whether this is helpful to the users in presenting, for example, new observations to them is the question. There will be such cases. But there will also be the opposite, where one is looking something up while one should be reading.

The above example is a special case of a general problem. What a researcher, in the practice of research, is able to make out of information by selecting, separating out, forgetting, letting insights ripen and mature, corresponds completely to what is to be found in the whole range of human practice. Information must be processed by selection, interpretation, evaluation. Where information comes within the reach of a person's practical consciousness, such processing will always be achieved in advance. The concept of information as applied by information theory in no way does justice to the process of selection through which an item of information becomes significant. Even the information on which the specialist builds up know-how through the logic of research is achieved 'hermeneutically'. This means that it is already limited to what it must answer by its questions. This is a hermeneutic structural element of all research. In itself it is still not 'practical' knowledge. All this is at once modified to the extent that the practical knowledge of human beings themselves becomes an object of science. This science is then no longer one which selects human beings themselves as the immediate object of its research. On the contrary, it takes up as its object *the knowledge* of human beings themselves which is mediated by the historical and cultural tradition. In Germany this is called, in the wake of the Romantic tradition, the *Geisteswissenschaften*.[11] The terms of other languages, such as 'humanities' or *lettres*, are clearer in so far as they convey the distinctiveness of the mode of givenness of the experience we actually encounter. In these sciences the logic of inquiry is in principle the same, indeed, as in every other science. But its object is something else. On the one hand, it is the human dimension which 'objectively' vouches for itself in the cultural creations of humankind such as economy, law, language, art and religion. On the other hand and in unison with this, its object is the explicit knowledge of humankind laid down in texts and verbal testaments.

The knowledge thus transmitted is indeed not of the type and status of the natural sciences. Nor is it a mere continuation beyond the borders of natural-scientific knowledge. Researchers into nature, deploring the absence of their exactness, may think unjustly of the humanities as 'inexact knowledge'. It may have the truth of vague intimations, which one calls understanding by introspection. In fact the teaching about humankind which we acquire through the *Geisteswissenschaften* is of an altogether different kind in which the immense variety of what is human manifests itself in its overwhelming breadth. The old differentiation made by the theory of knowledge between explanation and understanding or between nomothetic and idiographic methods does not suffice to indicate the full dimensions of a science of humankind that is self-conscious of its being a human activity. For what is manifest in concrete detail and belongs as such to historical knowledge is of interest not as the particular but as 'the human' – though it may always become visible only in particular occurrences. Everything human not only means the generally human in the sense of the characteristics of the human species in contrast to other types of living beings, especially animals, but also comprises the broad view of the variety of the human essence.

Without any doubt there is present here an unacknowledged idea of a norm in the light of which the fullness of the noticeable variations and deviations from what we expect from human beings and find valuable is articulated. All practical or political decisions which determine the actions of people are normatively determined and exert in their turn a norm-determining effect. Historical change is thus continually taking place. The knowledge which we owe to the results of research self-evidently plays a powerful role in this. But it is not a one-sided relationship. There are many mutual interactions between the human dimension as discovered scientifically through anthropological research and this intrinsically controversial and relative idea of value.

I am thinking not only of such facts as that researchers cannot always eliminate value expectations or that they will often interpret their findings under the impress of inappropriate prejudices – I am reminded again of the struggle over Darwinism in social research. These are at times overpowering defects in the progress of research. Similarly, researchers will not always be free of the inverted pleasure of discrediting established conceptions – this too will make them one-sided. But this is valid just as much in the positive. There are intuitive anticipations of knowledge, like the knowledge of salvation of the *homo religiosus*, which often has something to say to the doctor, or the 'knowledge' of the poet, which is able to outdistance that of the psychologist, sociologist, historian and philosopher. In short, the normative image of human beings, which, however incomplete and vague, lies at the basis of all human social behaviour, not only does not allow itself to be wholly eliminated in research but also should not be wholly eliminated. This is what makes science into an experience for human beings. All that the science of humankind can achieve in the attempt to bring about an integration of our knowledge of human beings is to unify both streams of knowledge and to make conscious the prejudices carried along by both. A 'correct' image of humankind is above all one which has been freed of dogmatism by natural science, research into behaviour, ethnology, as well as by the diversity of historical experience. It will be devoid of clear normative outlines if its scientific application relies on practice in the sense of 'social engineering'. As a critical standard, however, it frees people's actions from rash valuations, both positive and negative, and helps to remind us of the goal of the path of civilization which – left to its own resources – threatens to become less and less a path towards the advancement of humanity. It is thus that the science of humankind may serve people's self-knowledge and thereby practice.

Notes

This chapter was originally translated by Howard Brotz and has been modified by Jason Gaiger and Nicholas Walker.

1 Paul Natorp, *Philosophie, ihr Problem und ihre Probleme: Einführung in den kritischen Idealismus*, 3rd edn (Göttingen, 1921).
2 Benedetto Croce, *Logica come scienza del concetto puro* (Bari, 1905).
3 Jacob von Uexküll, *Streifzüge durch die Umwelten von Tieren und Menschen* (Frankfurt, 1970).
4 Philipp Lersch, *Die Binnenhaftigkeit des Seelischen* (Leipzig, 1941).
5 Arnold Gehlen, *Anthropologische Forschung* (Reinbek, 1961), and *Der Mensch*, 8th edn (Frankfurt, 1966).
6 Max Scheler, *Die Stellung des Menschen im Kosmos*, 7th edn (Munich, 1966).
7 Helmuth Plessner, *Philosophische Anthropologie* (Frankfurt, 1970).
8 Ibid.
9 Max Weber, 'Wissenschaft als Beruf', in his *Gesammelte Aufsätze zur Wissenschaftslehre*, 3rd edn (Tübingen, 1968).
10 Eliot Freidson, *Profession of Medicine: A Study of the Sociology of Applied Knowledge* (New York, 1970).
11 This term, which is commonly translated as 'human sciences' or 'cultural sciences', literally means, of course, 'sciences of the spirit'. It was coined, with its evident late Idealistic connotations, by the German translator of Mill's *Logic* to render thereby Mill's term 'moral sciences' (J. S. Mill, *System der deduktiven und induktiven Logik*, tr. Schied (1863), book 6: 'Von der Logik der Geisteswissenschaften oder moralischen Wissenschaften'). For a discussion of this term, see my paper 'The problem of historical consciousness', *Graduate Faculty Philosophy Journal*, vol. 5 (Fall 1975), p. 12.

2

Apologia for the Art of Healing

We still possess a treatise from the age of the Greek Sophists where we find the art of medicine defended against its detractors.[1] And it is certainly no accident that traces of a similar argument can be pursued even further back than this. For the art exercised in medicine is a strange one that does not correspond at every point with what the Greeks called *techne*, and what we call either applied art or science. The concept of *techne* is a peculiar creation of Greek culture, of the spirit of *historie*, the free-thinking investigation of things, and of the spirit of *logos*, the search for the explanatory grounds of everything we hold as true. The discovery of the concept of *techne* and its application to medicine marked a first decisive commitment towards everything that essentially characterizes western civilization. The physician no longer appears as the kind of medicine man mysteriously shrouded with special powers that we find in other cultures. He is a man with a body of knowledge. Aristotle specifically uses medicine as his standard example for the transformation of the purely practical accumulation of skill and knowledge into a genuine science. Even if the physician proves inferior to the experienced dispenser of cures or the wise old woman in a particular case, his knowledge possesses a fundamentally different character: he grasps the universal. He knows the reason why a particular form of healing meets with success. And he understands its effectiveness because he pursues the interconnection between cause and effect itself. That sounds very modern, and yet there is no question here of applying natural scientific knowledge to the practical goal of healing in our contemporary sense. For the opposition between pure science and its practical application as we are familiar with it has been shaped by the specific methods of modern science and the application of mathematics to the knowledge of nature. The Greek concept of *techne* on the other hand does not signify the practical application of theoretical knowing, but rather a special form of practical knowing. *Techne* is that knowledge which constitutes a specific and tried ability in the context of producing things. It is related from the very beginning to the sphere of production, and it is from this sphere that it first arose. But it represents a unique ability to produce, one which knows what it is doing, and knows on the basis of grounds. Thus it is a characteristic of this knowing ability from the outset that an *ergon*, or work, emerges from it and is released, as it were, from the activity of production. For production consummates itself in the fact that something independent is actually produced, that is, is given over for the use of others.

Now within the parameters of a concept of 'art' which still stands before the threshold of what we call 'science', it is obvious that the art of healing occupies an exceptional and problematic position. For here there is no 'work' produced by art, and no 'artificial' product. Here we cannot speak of a material which is already given in the last analysis by nature, and from which something new emerges by being brought into an artfully conceived form. On the contrary, it belongs to the essence of the art of healing that its ability to produce is an ability to re-produce and re-establish something. This signifies a special modification of what 'art' means, and one which is unique to the knowledge and practice of the physician. One can indeed say that physicians 'produce' health by means of their art, but this is not a very precise way of speaking. For what is produced in this way is not a work, an *ergon*, something quite new that comes into being and confirms the original skill. Rather it involves the restoration of the health of the sick person, and whether this is actually the result of medical knowledge and ability cannot be directly observed from the restored state of health itself. The healthy individual is not simply someone who has been 'made' healthy. Thus it must always remain an open question just how much the successful restoration of health owes to the experienced treatment of the physician and how much nature itself has assisted in the process.

This is the reason why from time immemorial there has always seemed something special about the art of medicine and the standing it enjoys. The literally vital significance of the art of medicine lends a particular status to physicians and their claims to knowledge and skill, especially when life is in mortal danger. On the other hand, and particularly when the danger is past, to this standing there always corresponds a certain doubt about the existence or the efficacy of such healing skills. *Tyche* and *techne*, fate and art, stand in a particularly tense and antagonistic relationship here. What is true for the positive case of successful healing is no less true for the negative case of failed treatment. What part was played by the negligence of the physician, we may ask, or was it perhaps the omnipotent stroke of fate which brought about the unlucky outcome? Who could decide such a thing, and especially those who do not possess the requisite skills? An apologia for the art of healing is more than a defence of a particular profession or a special art against other sceptical or unconvinced individuals; it also represents a kind of self-examination and self-defence on the part of the physician which indissolubly belongs to the peculiar character of medical skill itself. Physicians can no more prove the worth of their art to themselves than they can to others.

The characteristic ability which distinguishes the art of medicine in the context of *techne* stands, like all *techne*, within the broader context of nature. All ancient thought conceived the domain of what can skilfully be produced by human art in the light of nature. If *techne* was understood as the imitation of nature, then this principally signified that the artful capacity of human beings exploits and fills out, as it were, the open realm of possibilities which have been provided for us by the forms of nature itself. In this sense medicine is clearly not an imitation of nature, for there is no artificial product involved. What is supposed to emerge from the exercise of the physician's art is simply health, that is, nature itself. And this is what leaves its peculiar mark on the art of healing as a whole. It is not an art that involves the invention or planning of something new, of something which does not already exist as it is and which someone could go about producing in an instrumental fashion. On the contrary, it is from the beginning a particular kind of doing and making which produces nothing of its own and has no material of its own to produce something from. The expert practice of this art inserts itself entirely within the process of nature in so far as it seeks to restore this process when it is disturbed, and to do so in such a way that the art can allow itself to disappear once the natural equilibrium of health has returned. Physicians cannot stand back from their work in the way any artists, artisans or fabricators can, in such a way, that is, that they might in some sense retain the product as their own. Of course it is true in all cases of *techne* that the product is given over into the use of others, yet the product still remains one's own work. The work of physicians on the other hand, precisely because it is simply the health which has been restored, does not remain theirs in any way, and indeed it never was there. The relationship between the doing and the deed, the making and the made, the effort and the success is here of a fundamentally different, more enigmatic and elusive character.

In ancient medicine this can be seen among other things in the fact that an express effort had to be made to overcome the old temptation of only intervening and demonstrating one's skills where there was a chance of success. Even the individual who is fatally ill and who offers absolutely no hope of spectacular medical success still has to be an object of the doctor's concern, at least where there is a mature awareness among the medical profession, an awareness which goes hand in hand with philosophical insight into the *logos*. In this more profound sense the *techne* which is in question here is clearly integrated into the course of nature in such a way that it can make its contribution within the natural process as a whole and in all of its phases.

Now one can certainly recognize all these features in the modern science of medicine as well. And yet there has also been a fundamental transformation. For nature as the object of modern natural science is not the nature into which the medical skills, and indeed all the skills of human 'art', once felt themselves to be integrated. Indeed the peculiar character of the modern natural sciences lies in the fact that they understand their own knowledge precisely as a capacity to produce effects. The mathematical-quantitative isolation of laws and regularities in the natural order is directed towards the isolation of specific contexts of cause and effect which allow human action various possibilities for intervention which can be repeated under exact conditions. The concept of technology which is connected with the idea of science in the modern era thus takes on specifically intensified and increased possibilities in the field of medicine and its healing procedures. The capacity to produce desired effects makes itself independent, as it were. It permits the control of local physical processes and represents the application of a theoretical body of knowledge. As such, however, it is not a matter of healing, but rather of effecting something and so of producing something. In an area which is of vital interest to us all this pushes the division of labour proper to all social forms of human work to an extreme. The necessary integration of a differentiated body of knowledge and skills into the practical unity of treatment and healing cannot emerge from that powerful force of knowing and acting that modern science cultivates in a methodologically precise manner. Indeed, this is already an ancient article of wisdom that first appears in the mythological image of Prometheus and has found symbolic form for the entire European culture of the west in the figure of *Christus patiens*, namely the paradoxical injunction: 'Physician heal thyself.' But it is only in modern science that the acutely paradoxical character of all those procedures of *techne* so marked by the division of labour acquires its full and undiminished expression for the first time. The intrinsic impossibility of simply making oneself an object to oneself emerges completely only with the objectifying methods of modern science.

I should like to interpret the relationship at issue by recourse

to the concept of equilibrium and the way in which we experience it. This concept already plays a major role in the Hippocratic
writings. And in fact it is not merely the phenomenon of human
health which almost cries out to be understood in terms of the
natural condition of equilibrium. The concept of equilibrium also
readily offers itself for our understanding of nature in general.
The Greek concept of nature consisted in the discovery that the
totality is an ordered structure which allows all the processes of
nature to repeat themselves and to pass away in determinate
configurations. Nature is therefore something which as it were
holds to its own course, and does so in and of itself. This is the
fundamental idea of Ionian cosmology in which all the original
cosmogonic conceptions came to fulfilment: in the end the whole
mighty harmonious balance of interacting events determines all
things as a form of natural justice.[2]

If we presuppose this idea of nature, then medical intervention
must be understood as an attempt to restore an equilibrium that
has been disturbed. It is in this that the genuine 'work' of medical art consists. Let us ask ourselves therefore how the process
of re-producing such equilibrium is distinguished from every other
kind of producing. There is no doubt that this represents a quite
singular experience with which we are all familiar. We encounter
the recovery of equilibrium in exactly the same way as we encounter the loss of it, as a kind of sudden 'reversal'. Properly speaking
there is no continuous and perceptible transition from one to the
other, but rather a sudden change of state. This is quite different
from anything we are otherwise familiar with in the process of
production, where one brick is carefully laid down after another
and the change we are planning to effect is pursued step by step.
What we encounter here, by contrast, is the experience of balance, 'where the pure too little incomprehensibly transforms itself,
springs over into the empty too much.' That is how Rilke expresses
the phenomenon of balance as experienced by the acrobatic artist.
What he is describing is just this: the concentrated effort involved
in producing and maintaining equilibrium suddenly proves itself,
at the very moment when balance is attained, to be the opposite of what it seemed to be. For if the balancing act were to go

wrong, it would not be because physical force or power was lacking or too little was exerted, but rather because there was actually too much force in play. But when the act works, suddenly everything seems to happen spontaneously, lightly and effortlessly.

This experience can be seen to accompany every case where equilibrium is successfully produced. Those who strive to produce equilibrium find themselves thrown back, as it were, by something that is somehow self-sufficient and complete. Genuine success is accomplished in medical practice at just that point where intervention is ultimately rendered superfluous and dispensable. All medical efforts at healing are already conceived from the outset in light of the fact that the doctor's contribution consummates itself by disappearing as soon as the equilibrium of health is restored. In our experience of balance the exertion involved is paradoxically directed at somehow loosening its own grip, precisely in order to allow equilibrium itself to come into play; but all our medical exertions possess a similar inner relationship to the process in which nature itself comes into play. The ultimate horizon of all medical practice is defined by the fact that the fluctuating state of equilibrium characteristic of health is qualitatively distinct from that definitive loss of equilibrium when everything finally comes to an end.

But the consequence to be drawn from this is that medical practice is not concerned with actually producing equilibrium, that is, with building up a new state of equilibrium from nothing, but rather is always concerned with arresting and assisting the fluctuating equilibrium of health. All disturbance of this equilibrium, all sickness, still takes place against the background of incontestable factors directly connected with the ongoing general equilibrium of the body. And that is the reason why the doctor's intervention cannot properly be understood simply as making or effecting something, but must rather principally be seen as a case of supporting those factors that help to sustain equilibrium. Medical intervention always stands under a double sign: the act of intervening either constitutes a disturbing factor itself or it introduces a specific healing effect into the play of harmoniously interacting factors. It seems to me to be constitutive for the essence of the doctor's art that it must always reckon in advance with the potential 'reversal' of the too much into the too little, or rather of the too little into the too much, and try as it were to anticipate it.

And here our ancient text on the art of healing offers us a beautiful example with the practice of tree-sawing. As one partner draws the blade the other follows in concert, so that the whole sawing process constitutes what Viktor von Weiszäcker calls a *Gestaltkreis*, an internally unified configuration in which the respective movements of the two tree-cutters fuse to become a single rhythmic flux of movement. And here we come on a significant remark which suggests something of the mysterious character of equilibrium: 'Yet if they employ violent force, then they will fail utterly.' This insight is certainly not confined to the art of healing, for all mastery in productive craft knows something of this. The skilled hand of the master lets the deed appear effortless in just the place where the apprentice produces only a forced effect. Every practised skill possesses something of this experience of equilibrium. But the peculiar character of the art of medicine lies in the fact that it is not concerned here with the total mastery of a skill that is demonstrated directly by producing an accomplished piece of work. Hence the particular solicitude of the doctor who must continue to respect the equilibrium which persists in spite of all disturbance and must stay attuned to the natural process of that equilibrium, just like the tree-cutter in our example.

If we now relate this fundamental experience to the situation of modern science and scientific medicine, it emerges very clearly just how and why the whole problem has become so acute. Modern natural science is not primarily a science of nature conceived as a self-maintaining and self-restoring totality. Our science is based not on the experience of life but on that of making and producing, not on the experience of equilibrium but on that of projective construction. This science is essentially – going far beyond the domain of that special science which bears the name – a kind of mechanics: it is *mechane*, that is, the artificial production of effects which would not come about simply of themselves.

Originally the Greek term merely designated some significant invention that aroused the astonishment of all. But a modern science facilitating technological application does not understand itself as something that steps in to occupy the open domain yielded by nature itself or as something that must integrate itself into the entire process of nature. Rather it understands itself precisely as a kind of knowledge that is guided by the idea of transforming nature into a human world, indeed almost of eliminating the natural dimension by means of rationally controlled projective 'construction'. As science this knowledge allows us to calculate and to control natural processes to such an extent that it finally becomes capable of *replacing* the natural by the artificial. This lies in the very essence of science. For the application of mathematics and quantitative methods generally within the natural sciences is only possible because the knowledge involved is a form of construction. But our reflections have already taught us that the art of healing remains ineliminably bound up with the presupposition that was still implied in the ancient concept of nature. Among all the sciences concerned with nature the science of medicine is the one which can never be understood entirely as a technology, precisely because it invariably experiences its own abilities and skills simply as a restoration of what belongs to nature. And that is why medicine represents a peculiar unity of theoretical knowledge and practical know-how within the domain of the modern sciences, a unity moreover which as such cannot be understood as the application of science to the field of praxis. Medicine itself represents a peculiar kind of practical science for which modern thought no longer possesses an adequate concept.

In the light of these reflections there is a beautiful and much discussed passage in Plato's *Phaedrus* (270b ff.) which acquires a special interest for us since it illuminates the predicament of the physician who possesses this 'science'. Plato speaks here about the true art of rhetoric and draws a parallel with the art of healing. For in both cases it is a question of understanding nature, either the nature of the soul or the nature of the body, at least if we are hoping to act on grounds of genuine knowledge rather than merely on the basis of routine and everyday experience. Just as we must know which remedies and what sustenance should be administered to the body if it is to become healthy and vigorous once again, so too one must know which laws and ordinances and which kinds of discourse should be introduced to the soul, if it is to acquire the proper convictions and attain its authentic being or virtue (*arete*). Socrates turns to his young friend who is so inspired by the feats of rhetoric and asks: 'Do you believe that one can understand the nature of the soul without understanding the nature of the whole?' And his friend replies: 'If we may believe Hippocrates the Asclepiad, then one cannot even understand anything of the body without this procedure' (Phdr. 270c). The two conceptual moments of the 'nature of the whole' and 'this procedure' (namely that of dividing and distinguishing phenomena within nature) obviously belong together. The true craft of rhetoric which is demanded by Socrates here will resemble the true art of medicine in so far as it must also be familiar with the manifold nature of the soul in which it wishes to implant the proper convictions, and familiar with the manifold kinds of discourse which are appropriate for the constitution of the particular soul in question. This is the analogy which is developed with an eye to the activities and skills of the physician. The true art of healing, which involves an authentic knowing and doing, thus requires the capacity to distinguish between the particular constitution of the organism in question and what is actually compatible with that constitution.

In interpreting this passage Werner Jaeger rightly rejected the idea that Plato was here demanding a special type of medical art inspired by a specific philosophy of nature and universal cosmological conceptions. Quite the opposite is the case. The procedure at issue is that of 'division': a differentiating examination of the various manifestations of sickness with a view to grasping a specific unified picture of the sickness in question, which will then permit us to pursue an integrated course of treatment. It is well known that the concept of *eidos* or form which is familiar to us from the Platonic doctrine of ideas was actually first employed in the context of medical knowledge. Thus we encounter it in Thucydides in his account of the disease induced by the famous plague which befell Athens at the beginning of the Peloponnesian war and which eventually also claimed Pericles as its victim. And in all its re-searches medical science has been guided even to the present day by the same demand. This method of division is actually anything but a scholastic exercise in conceptual hair-splitting. Division here does not imply the isolation of a particular part from the context of the whole. Socrates forbids the purely isolated examination of symptoms and precisely thereby demands real scientific knowledge. But in this connection Socrates goes beyond what modern medical science recognizes as its methodological basis. The nature of the whole that is at issue here is not merely the unified whole of the single organism. We possess abundant evidence from Greek medicine to show us how the weather and the seasons, how tem-perature, water and general sustenance, in short how all possible climatic and environmental factors were seen to make up the concrete ontological constitution of what it is that the physician helps to restore, namely health. But the context in which this passage stands also permits a further conclusion to be drawn. The nature of the whole includes and involves the entire life situation of the patient, and even of the physician. Medicine is compared with the true art of rhetoric which allows the right kinds of discourse to exercise an effect on the soul in the right kinds of way.

This is a highly ironic manner of depicting things. For Plato is certainly not envisaging an art of rhetoric suitable for guiding the soul, one which would be able to instil and to exploit any kind of discourse for any arbitrary purpose whatsoever. On the con-trary, he obviously means that only the right kinds of discourse may be involved, and that only someone who has seen the truth can recognize what the right kinds of discourse are. The only individual capable of being the right kind of rhetorical speaker will be the true philosopher and practitioner of dialectic. But the art of medicine which has been compared with that of rhetoric is now placed in an extremely interesting light. Just as the appar-ently specific tasks of rhetoric must be integrated into the whole philosophical way of life, so too something similar is the case with all those means of treatment which medicine applies to the human body in the hope of restoring its health. The parallel between the art of rhetoric and the art of medicine is also valid to the extent that the constitution of the body passes over into the constitution of the human being as a whole. The position of the human individual within the totality of being is a balancing position not merely in the sense of stably maintained health but also in a much more comprehensive sense. For sickness, and loss of equilibrium, do not merely represent a medical-biological state of affairs, but also a life-historical and social process. The sick person is no longer simply identical with the person he or she was before. For the sick individual 'falls out' of things, has already fallen out of their normal place in life. But the individual who now lacks and misses something previously enjoyed still remains orientated towards returning to that former life. If the restoration of natural equilibrium is successfully accomplished, then the miraculous process of convalescence also returns the healthy back into the general equilibrium of the life in which they were formerly active and could be themselves. Thus it is not so strange that the reverse is also true and that the loss of one kind of equilibrium always endangers the other kind at the same time, that indeed in the last analysis there is only one single great equilibrium which sustains human life and which, though it sometimes wavers and flickers, fundamentally determines our very state of being.

In this sense Plato's suggestion that the physician, like the true rhetorician, must take the whole of nature into view remains valid. Just as the latter must draw on true insight to find the right word which will influence those who listen, so too the physician must look beyond the immediate object of his knowledge and skill if he is to be a true physician. The position of doctors thus remains a fragile and intermediate one between enjoying a particular professional existence just like any other, with no special human commitments, and participating in something that is binding upon our very humanity. The predicament of doctors is defined by their capacity for inspiring trust but also and equally by the necessity of limiting the use of their professional power and influence. Doctors must be able to look beyond the 'case' they are treating and have regard for the human being as a whole in that person's particular life situation. Indeed doctors must even be capable of reflecting on their own medical intervention and its probable effect on the patient. They must know when to stand back. For they must neither make patients wholly dependent on them, nor needlessly prescribe dietary or other conditions of lifestyle which would only hinder patients from returning to their own equilibrium of life.

What is generally recognized to hold in respect of the relationship between the psychiatrist and the mentally ill, and as constituting the accepted task of the psychotherapist, must also be recognized to possess a more universal validity. The doctor's art ultimately consists in withdrawing itself and helping to set the other person free. Here too the peculiar position which the art of healing enjoys among all the other arts emerges with particular clarity. Anyone who exercises a particular art or skill finds a certain limitation imposed on them by the fact that the fabricated product of their art is detached from its process of origin and given over into the free use of others. But in the case of the doctor this becomes a genuine instance of self-limitation. For the doctor has not simply brought about a special piece of work that he or she has actually made. Rather the doctor has been entrusted with a human life which must now be released from this protective care. And the individual patient is in a corresponding situation. Those who have regained health and been given back to their own life begin to forget the illness, but still remain bound and beholden to the doctor in a specific, if often unspoken, manner.

Notes

1 Translated into German as *Die Apologie der Heilkunst*, ed., trans., annotated and introduced by Theodor Gomperz, Sitzungsbericht der Kaiserlichen Akademie der Wissenschaften in Wien (Vienna, 1890).
2 On the question of cosmological justice see the only surviving fragment of Anaximander, VS 12 A 9: 'and the source of coming-to-be for existing things is that into which destruction, too, happens "according to necessity"; for they pay penalty and retribution to each other for their injustice according to the

assessment of Time' (in *The Presocratic Philosophers*, trans. G. S. Kirk and J. E. Raven (Cambridge, 1957), p. 106). See also my essay 'Platon und die Vorsokratiker', in H.-G. Gadamer, *Gesammelte Werke* (Tübingen, 1985–), vol. 6, pp. 58–70, esp. pp. 62ff.

3

The Problem of Intelligence

The philosopher is interested in the problems of science from a curiously inverted perspective. And this is also the case with the problem of intelligence. While doctors or psychologists employ the concept of intelligence in a specific manner that is clearly defined by the phenomena described, the philosopher asks how the concept of intelligence has already been shaped as such, and enquires after the prior articulation of the world of experience implicitly contained in the concept itself. In both scientific and everyday language use the concept of intelligence is one which is appropriately employed to measure performance: it expresses a general ability which is not determined by any particular capacity or by its relation to any particular objects of thought. In the living use of language, words never exist in isolation. Their meaning is sustained and determined through the proximity and influence of neighbouring words. If we look at our current use of language to see which words are closely allied to the concept of intelligence – neighbouring expressions such as astuteness, rapid mental grasp, cleverness in general or the power of judgement – then we can see that they share the same formal structure as the concept of intelligence. At the same time, however, they are not identical with it. Thus the first question which the philosopher must ask is whether the characterization of such a formal concept of intelligence does not itself already reflect a prior decision, not to say a prejudgement about the issue.

Some historical reflections may serve to clarify the legitimacy of this question further. It seems that the meaning of the word 'intelligence' as we know it is of relatively recent date. In the language both of philosophy and of the psychology which was influenced by it, the classical Latin word originally held a very different place. *Intelligentia* referred to the highest form of insight, superior even to *ratio*, the rational use of concepts and forms of thought. *Intelligentia* is the Latin philosophical equivalent to the Greek concept *nous*, which we normally, and not so inaccurately, render as 'reason' or even 'spirit'. Primarily it denotes the ability to recognize and identify the highest principles. However, the use of language which is prevalent today is separated from this philosophical prehistory of the word *intelligentia* by a caesura. It is not easy to characterize this break with any exactness. The concept of intelligence as we use it today was still quite unknown in the philosophical psychology of the eighteenth century. However, to a certain extent linguistic usage, in particular the French adjective *intelligent*, already current in the fifteenth century, did anticipate the formal definition of this new concept of intelligence. The new way of defining this concept has significant consequences and shows what sort of prior conceptual decisions are sedimented in concepts. The fact that in the seventeenth century *intelligence* ceased to refer to the capacity to know principles and began to mean the general ability to recognize things, facts, relations, etc., placed man on essentially the same plane as the intelligent animals. Clearly it was the Enlightenment which, motivated by pragmatic ideals, separated the concept of intelligence from any relation to principles and began to apply it purely instrumentally. In connection with current language use, which was developing in a pragmatic direction, the Enlightenment aimed to avoid the extreme consequences of Cartesianism, which had reserved self-consciousness for humankind and defined animals simply as machines. One can see that our contemporary concept of intelligence received its formal character from a particular set of questions which in no way directly corresponds to the original field of meaning which belonged to the Latin word *intelligentia*.

This suspicion is further reinforced if we look back at the conceptuality of Greek philosophy and ask what might there properly correspond to our concept of 'intelligence'. It can with justice be claimed that the Greeks in fact possess no philosophical concept which represents a real equivalent to our own. Of course, in the Greek language of the classical age, and even in the time of Homer, there are linguistic equivalents for characterizing someone as intelligent, such as the cunning and resourceful Odysseus, or words which refer to the power of understanding (for example, *synesis*). However, Greek philosophy never developed a formal concept of intelligence. Should this fact not be taken into account? If the Greeks compared the phenomenon, so disconcerting to us, of animal behaviour which although guided by instinct is still apparently 'intelligent' with the intelligent behaviour of human beings, it none the less seems to me significant that the concept with which they made this comparison, that of *phronesis*, also possessed a completely different substantial meaning which belongs in the human realm of moral philosophy. Thus, for example, Aristotle claimed that certain animals also clearly possess *phronesis*. He was thinking primarily about bees and ants, about animals which gather food for the winter and so, from a human point of view, reveal foresight, something which must include an awareness of time. An awareness of time – this is something momentous. For it does not signify merely an increase in knowledge, in the power of anticipation, but involves what is in fact a fundamentally different status altogether. It means the ability to forgo the gratification of the most immediate goal in favour of a long-term fixed purpose.

The concept of *phronesis* is thus applied to animal behaviour on the basis of an analogy with human behaviour, but in the moral and human domain Aristotle especially gave it a precise definition which should give us cause for thought. Aristotle was able to follow closely current linguistic usage, that sedimented reason which resides in all use of language. He considered *phronesis* not only as the clever, skilful discovery of means for meeting specific tasks, not only as an awareness of what is practical, of how to realize incidental goals, but also as the sense for setting the goals themselves and taking responsibility for them. The concept of *phronesis* thereby acquires, and this is what is important, a substantive determination. This concept does not denote a merely formal capacity, but rather includes at the same time a further determination, namely its field of application. On one occasion Aristotle expresses this by contrasting *phronesis* with *deinotes*; he opposes the exemplary bearing of *phronesis* to its naturally contrasting opposite, the uncanny skilfulness which is able to master every possible situation – and this is not at all something which is held to be wholly positive. Anyone who possesses this capacity is, as we say, capable of anything and is able, where it is exercised without reservation or any sense of responsibility, to win from every situation a practical advantage and to profit from it. (In politics, for example, this is the unprincipled exponent of expediency, in economic life the financial opportunist who is not to be trusted, and in the social realm it is the confidence trickster.)

The concept of intelligence, then, seems here still to be bound up with the totality of what it is to be human, with our *humanitas*. Just like the familiar concept of sound common sense, it seems to have lost an essential dimension in modern thought. In general we do not think that sound common sense could be anything other than a merely formal capacity (the normal endowment with an ability) and yet when we examine this concept more closely we can see that it possesses a quite different meaning. It corresponds, in fact, to the French concept of *bon sens* and, ultimately, to the notion of *sensus communis*, that is, common sense as public spirit. It can be shown that *sensus communis*, common sense, does not in fact mean only the undisturbed use of our mental faculties, but always at the same time possesses a substantial content.[1] *Sensus communis* as common sense does not refer only to that *facultas dijudicativa* which processes the evidence of the particular senses; it refers primarily to that social sense, to that public spiritedness which contains certain commonly shared and undisputed substantial assumptions; it is in no way merely the formal ability to make use of our faculty of reason.

This seems to me significant for our considerations concerning the concept of intelligence and its original connection with the concept of *intelligentia*. The scientific legitimation for detaching the concept of intelligence from the specific substantial problems that we face as human beings is neither self-evident nor beyond question. If we ask ourselves what such a detachment really means we must first and fundamentally reflect on the fact that every concept of this type contains a specific, socially determined conventional character, a particular, socially established normative meaning. Society comprehends itself in the living character of its use of language and it says something about itself when it uses particular expressions such as 'intelligence' in the way with which we are familiar. How then does our society understand itself and what does it intend by this concept? Is it perhaps something more than a contingent linguistic fact that our familiar concept of intelligence is of such recent date?

With this I do not wish to repeat the well-known critique of so-called faculty psychology. It is true that with the concept of 'faculty' the classical psychology of the eighteenth century articulated a specific fundamental conception of human beings and their abilities and that the abandonment of this apparatus of faculties with which the soul was supposedly equipped was indisputably important in furthering our knowledge of human existence. 'Intelligence' as it is employed in current linguistic usage is clearly not a faculty in the sense intended by classical psychology. This means that 'intelligence' is not used today to refer to just one of the functions or forms of activity of the human mind, which as a specifically mental function might either be brought into play or not, alongside other functions like those of the senses for example. Rather, intelligence is present in all human behaviour. Or, to put it another way, in all intelligent behaviour the entire person is present. It is a way of life in which each person situates himself or herself; it is so constitutive of our being human at all that we do not have that distance towards it which would enable us to choose whether to pursue it or not to pursue it, to bring it into play or not to do so.

Even if this is conceded, the construction of the concept of 'intelligence' as we now use it may none the less still retain something from the old, superseded stage of faculty psychology. What I mean is this: the fact that today we largely conceive intelligence as a formal concept for measuring performance turns it, in a certain sense, into a tool or instrument. For it is the determining characteristic of a tool that it signifies nothing in its own right but is rather simply something suited for the manifold range of uses in which it is employed. It is perhaps a special tool that is denoted by the term intelligence, by our faculty of intelligence, or however we choose to express it; it is special by virtue of its universality, because unlike other tools it is not limited to a particular use and suitable only for a specific application. But it does not seem to me superfluous to ask whether the concept of an instrument, of a tool made for use, which is necessarily involved in the now accepted formal concept of intelligence does not reveal a questionable understanding of human beings and a questionable concept of intelligence.[2]

In comparison with the naive self-evidence with which the concept of instinct or of purposeful machines was once elucidated by reference to the notion of human self-consciousness, all our reflections today about people and animals or about people and machines share one thing in common, namely a scepticism about the claims of self-consciousness which has become unavoidable since Nietzsche. Where Descartes saw self-consciousness as the *fundamentum inconcussum* of all certainty, Nietzsche came up with the motto: 'We must doubt even more fundamentally.'[3] Indeed, the concept of the unconscious has opened up an entirely new dimension which leaves self-consciousness with a merely epiphenomenal sphere of legitimacy. Yet to a large extent the philosophy of the modern age was grounded on the indubitability of self-consciousness. The concept of reflection in particular, indispensable to us for determining the various phenomena of the mind, rests on this ground. Reflection, the free process of turning in on oneself, appears as the highest form of freedom that exists at all. Here the mind is properly in its own element in so far as it relates solely to its own content. It is undeniable that this freedom in relation to oneself, this original distance, does characterize an essential feature of being human. Moreover, it is also true that some sort of ability to stand back from oneself is a fundamental prerequisite for linguistic orientation in the world, and in this sense all reflection is in fact freedom.

None the less, in light of the critique of self-consciousness which characterizes modernity, it would seem rather dubious to speak of an elevation into the realm of the mind, as if we were capable of raising ourselves up into and moving freely within this dimension through a free act of decision. Perhaps there are many different forms of reflection. In any case, in every ability there resides some form of reflection. It is constitutive of the concept of an ability that it is not merely the performance of an action but, in contrast to every such potential performance, also means the prior possession of this possibility. Thus it is part of the consciousness which is proper to all genuine ability that it involves mastery over the application of its own skill. Plato showed that he was already aware of this inner reflexivity in the concept of ability (*techne*) when he stressed that every ability is at the same time the ability both to do something and to do its opposite.[4] Thus the person who is truly skilled at running is the one who can run both slowly and quickly. The person who is truly skilled at lying is the one who knows both what is true and what is false, and for this reason, in wishing to lie, is careful not to tell the truth by accident. This concept of ability implies a certain distance towards the performance of the act involved; it is thus principally determined by that structure which we call reflexivity. However, is this reflection which resides in the 'free ability' of *techne* the right model for the essential reflexivity which is characteristic of human beings? It really remains an open question whether human beings are capable of such free elevation into a critical distance from themselves and whether this elevation into the realm of the mind, into the realm of self-consciousness, lifts them out of the constraints of their finitude and actuality.

In the striking and astute discussion of the concept of dementia which Zutt has presented[5] this question becomes pressing at just the point where he characterizes extreme forms of dementia in terms of the patients' lack of awareness that they are ill. This is doubtless descriptively true, and yet it touches on a fundamental problem. What does it mean to say that someone is aware that they are ill? It is clearly a misrepresentation of the phenomenon to look at the concept of illness solely through the eyes of the doctor and from the standpoint of scientific medicine, and to think that medical knowledge is the same thing as the patient's own self-understanding. As a phenomenon of lived experience, insight into one's own illness is clearly not simply insight in the sense of knowledge of a true state of affairs, but rather, like all insight, it is something which is acquired with great difficulty and by overcoming significant resistance. We know the important role which concealment of the awareness of ill-health plays in certain human illnesses and, above all, what an important part this concealment can play in the lived existence of a person.

The patient experiences his or her illness through the felt absence of something. What does this absence of something tell us; what does it tell us about that which is missing? It must occasion reflection that extreme cases of dementia are incompatible with an awareness of being ill, that often even the initial stages are closed off to such awareness. It is no doubt an uncontroversial scientific observation to recognize that someone in a condition which science characterizes as illness – in comparision with a conception of normal health – has lost the ability to take up a certain distance towards themselves and to recognize that they are ill, and perhaps even that a certain type of illness consists in the loss of the ability to take up such a position of distance towards oneself. However, the establishment of such an extreme condition does not exclude the question of whether the capacity for reflection, the ability to take up a certain distance towards oneself, is not a necessary condition of all mental illness. And one can also ask whether, for the patients themselves, insight into their own illness, or the lack of such insight, means nothing more than insight into the factual presence of something.

In fact, the necessity of doubting with Nietzsche the evidence of consciousness can be confirmed through reference to several concrete forms of self-consciousness, such as self-criticism, including cultural criticism, and, ultimately, the phenomenon of insight into one's own ill-health.[6] If we are not to fall into a form of naive dogmatism, we cannot simply presuppose that insight into what exists is an open possibility for human beings, that this is an essential determining characteristic of their being, a standpoint of critical distance to which they can at all times raise themselves. In ways that are difficult to describe, the capacity to gain insight and to acquire critical distance remains bound up with the individual person in the totality of their life situation. True, it is characteristic of human beings, as opposed to the remarkable abilities and skills possessed by creatures such as bees, beavers, ants and spiders, that they are aware of their own abilities and therefore possess the astonishing capacity of 'deliberately' refraining from the exercise of their acquired skills under particular circumstances, that is, of demonstrating their freedom even in respect to their technical arts. However, such freedom is, like the capacity for reflective distance in general, something problematic. To pursue this freedom is not itself in turn a free act but is rather something motivated, with conditions and intentional grounds which are not themselves under the control of the free exercise of one's ability. Thus it is only a formal analogy to compare such ability with a tool, an instrument which is simply taken up at will or set aside. Every ability is a mode of being.

This is the reason why the structure of reflection is not always bound up with the notion of objectification. One's own self, of which one can become reflexively conscious, is not an object in the same sense as something normally grasped in the objectifying attitude which knowledge adopts towards an object. Such an object, as soon as it is known, loses its power of resistance, is conquered and becomes disposable. *Natura parendo vincitur* ('we conquer nature by obeying her'). Reflection, as the capacity to take up a certain distance towards oneself, is not the same as a relation of opposition towards an object. Reflection is rather brought into play in such a way that it accompanies the lived performance of a task. This is our real freedom, which enables choices and decisions to be made even as we participate in the performance of life itself. There is no other freedom, no condition into which we are able to elevate ourselves through a free act of decision. What properly belongs to an action which we call 'intelligent' is just this capacity to sustain reflection along with the performance of a task, and not any sort of objectifying confrontation.

What this means, and this is the moment of 'reflection', is that the immediacy of access to something is broken; as Hegel would put it, desire is held in check and it is precisely thereby that we become conscious of the goal as such. The desire is recognized as something unattained and is thus posited as a 'goal'. To this extent consciousness is in fact consciousness of a disturbance. Wolfgang Köhler's account of his experiments with monkeys provides a good illustration of this. The frustrated desire for a banana leads to a certain 'thoughtfulness', that is, when the desire remains fixed on its goal it leads to an indirect recourse to something else, to something that is not itself a goal, but rather a means to an end. But such a 'means to an end' is not really itself an object of attention, any more than one's own hand becomes an 'object' when it is unable to reach what is desired simply by stretching out. Rather, this 'attention' and the thoughtfulness which is both directed towards attaining the goal and yet turned away from it are expressed in the action of achieving the goal; once the goal is achieved the means which were formerly 'at hand' are cast aside. The disturbance requires the removal of what is causing the interference, that is, it requires the eventual disappearance of attention to oneself.

I consider this to be the model through which all self-reflection must be understood, especially that form of reflection which is involved in the awareness of one's own ill-health. Here too it is not a matter of taking up an objectifying attitude towards oneself in such a way that the illness can be 'established'. Rather, one is thrown back on oneself because something is felt to be lacking, because there is a disturbance which is already orientated towards finding a resolution, even if this· is to be achieved by submitting oneself to the diagnosis and intervention of a doctor. Illness is, in the last analysis, not the established result which scientific medicine declares as illness but, rather, the experience of the person suffering it. It is that experience which, just like every other disturbance, the individual seeks to bring to an end.

Illness, then, is in general experienced by the person who is ill as a disturbance which can no longer be ignored. The recognition that something is lacking is connected with the idea of balance, and this means in particular with the idea of a restoration of equilibrium out of all the fluctuating conditions that constitute an individual's general state of health. Within this context illness represents a fall from a self-sustaining equilibrium into a state of unbalance. This must be kept in mind wherever the role of the patient's awareness of their own illness becomes a problem. It is part of the balancing act of life that one learns to forget what is causing a disturbance, or at least succeeds in regarding it with indifference. One of the means for sustaining this skill of balancing is precisely intelligent behaviour, including, for example, self-deception or the knowing refusal to accept the truth of one's own illness. For illness as the loss of health, as the loss of one's un-disturbed 'freedom', always involves a sort of exclusion from 'life'. It is for this reason that awareness of ill-health represents a problem which affects someone's life as a whole and which concerns the whole person. Such awareness is by no means a free act of intelligence, the adoption of a critical distance and the objectification of oneself and the experienced disturbance. Everything the doctor identifies in the 'difficult' patient, the resistance against the doctor and the patient's refusal to accept their own condition of need and powerlessness, all this belongs to the sphere of illness as a problem which affects life as a whole. This situation is evidence precisely of a level of intelligence which finds it difficult to submit to medical authority. Whether in the form of insight or of a blind lack of insight, reflection here does not involve a free turning of attention towards oneself. Rather it remains permanently under the pressure of suffering, of the will to life, of the fixation on work, profession, prestige or whatever.

The intervention of the doctor does not fundamentally change anything in this situation. The patient enters into the new life situation which had made the awareness of ill-health necessary.

The doctor is there to help, indeed to help re-establish the lost equilibrium. It is particularly the practitioners of modern medicine who are aware that this means not merely overcoming somatic problems, but rather bringing back into proper balance the life situation of the disorientated patient who has lost control over it. Thus medical intervention, in the very act of helping, is always in danger of disturbing the equilibrium once again. It can do so not only through 'dangerous' operations which disturb other delicate relations of balance, but also by placing the patient within a vast and incomprehensible network of psychological and social difficulties.

If we address the problem of mental illness from this perspective and raise the question of what role intelligence plays here, then it is quite clear that mental illness, of whatever sort, represents a loss of equilibrium. And we can ask how far this loss affects that intelligent behaviour which facilitates insight into one's own illness. The common usage of the concept of intelligence can easily lead us into confusion here so that we fail to recognize that an ill 'mind' does not by any means need to suffer any decline in intelligence. For this reason Langer's report on the particularly high degree of intelligence generally possessed by neurotics was very instructive. If illness is characterized as a loss of equilibrium then it is easy to accept that the formal faculty which we call intelligence can be quite independent of the general mental state of someone who is ill. For by the expression 'general mental state' we do not understand a formal faculty but rather everything which someone has in mind, what ideas they have, what order of values they are governed by, what essential goals they set before themselves and how these sustain or disrupt the equilibrium of their lives. That there are forms of illness in which 'intelligence', as the capacity for reflective distance, is completely extinguished should lead us perhaps to identify the heart of the matter in terms of the disintegration of a human person, rather than of the loss of any formal faculty. The equilibrium which we call mental health is precisely a condition of the person as a whole being who is not simply a bundle of capacities; such equilibrium concerns the totality of a person's whole relation to the world.

Admittedly it can be objected that it is not for nothing that we speak of 'mental' illness. What does 'the mind' mean here? Does it not always include the capacity to adopt a free relationship to oneself, to achieve a certain distance from oneself, to participate in the intellectual dimension in general? This question forces itself on us with renewed urgency if, starting out from a consideration of the intelligent behaviour of animals, one seeks to determine what is specific to human intelligence. The human being is the creature who possesses language. For the linguistic character of our relationship to the world is undoubtedly closely bound up with the nature of our intelligence. If one begins by considering our lived situation and our attempts to master or direct it, then this intellectual or spiritual dimension may come to seem like another dimension altogether. The mind or spirit can be seen, if not as some sort of antagonist to life, then at least as the expression of an internal disintegration within life itself, one in which we no longer unquestioningly follow the accustomed paths but rather develop a world mediated by our own independent thought. We thus represent to ourselves a linguistically interpreted world where we are surrounded by possibilities among which we must choose. This ability to choose could be interpreted simply as a means which is both fitting and necessary for the achievement of a particular goal, the self-preservation and good health of humankind. The naturalness of language seems to attest to this: it is the most intellectual and spiritual of all means of gaining understanding. To that extent intelligence would also be such a 'means', something that enables human beings to cope successfully with their existence. Its failure to function appropriately in the case of illness would surely represent, as with any other disease, simply a breakdown, differing only according to its degree of severity, even to the point where any recognition of one's own state of illness has become impossible.

But it is just this account that is inadequate. For what fundamentally characterizes the essential constitution of human beings is that although their nature, just like that of any other living being, strives after fulfilment, what counts for them as fulfilment is not unquestioningly pre-established; rather, they can set their own goals for themselves. The diverse range of possibilities towards which they can orientate themselves and among which they can choose are forms of self-interpretation which correspond to the interpretation of the world through language. In my opinion, Aristotle judged rightly when he allowed our sense for what is beneficial and what is harmful to pass over into our sense for what is 'right' or 'just'. For it is this which characterizes human-kind as the *zoon logon exon* ('the living being that possesses discourse') in contrast to the immediacy of animal desire.[7] Language, which is able to express both senses, is not simply a means of understanding adaptable to contingent ends. Language does not merely serve us in promoting what is beneficial and avoiding what is harmful. It is what first establishes common goals and makes them into something we are responsible for; goals through which human beings by nature give form to their social existence.

Here there is, of course, 'distance', but this distance with respect to various possibilities is what is closest to us as human beings, it is the distance within which we live. There is no objective field for neutral observation here. Rather, these human potentialities belong, like the world itself, to that whole in which the task of learning to be 'at home', of establishing oneself, is precisely what living means for man. Human life is threatened by illness, that is, by the loss of equilibrium, and since it is a human life this loss of equilibrium is always one which affects the whole of the person, which affects psychological balance as well. It is most fully and evidently in the area where the doctor speaks of 'mental' illness that we encounter loss of equilibrium. That we can no longer cope with being surrounded by possibilities represents a breakdown in our capacity to sustain psychological self-balance. This breakdown is not independent of the horizon of the possibilities which surround us, no matter whether they help to sustain the state of equilibrium in which we find ourselves or whether they contribute to destroying it through our ecstatic self-abandonment and fixation on one particular possibility. Such dangers as these are not to be encountered in the instinctive features of the animal life-world. What intelligence means there, or seems to mean, is an intelligent mode of obeying instinct, that is, a form of behaviour orientated towards attaining predetermined goals. Human intelligence, on the other hand, concerns the setting of the goals themselves and the choice of the right form of life (*bios*). It is not merely a capacity for skilful adaptation, resourcefulness and mental agility in the meeting of pre-given tasks; in this even the psychopath can be superior to the 'healthy' person. There is here a specific methodological aporia which affects all attempts to test intelligence. Such tests always confront the candidate with tasks, no matter how well disguised, which the candidate has not chosen and is aware of not having chosen. Thus it seems to me a fundamental impoverishment of the process of concept formation when we seek to define the concept of human intelligence through direct analogy with that of animals.

For this is to consider the human person in terms of the instinctual forces which are proper to animal forms of life. Animal 'intelligence' betrays something quite different than in the case of human beings, for whom the constraints of instinct are transformed through a powerful institutionalization of cultural forms. For humankind, intelligence must possess a wholly different meaning. The formal concept of intelligence unintentionally allows the human person to be used as a tool, to be treated as a manipulable collection of capacities, whose maximal suitability for established goals defines the normative social concept of intelligence. To say that 'someone belongs to the class of intelligent people' is to refer to their sociopolitical qualification, their suitability for government purposes in the eyes of the authorities responsible for direction and planning. In the end we are astonished to discover that talk of the intelligence of animals is not in fact a dubious form of *anthropomorphism*. Rather, the way we commonly talk of the intelligence of human beings, one which is informed by the normative ideal of a measurable quota of intelligence, represents a secret and unacknowledged *theriomorphism*.

For me the importance of psychiatry lies in its ability to counteract this tendency by drawing on the experience of what is involved in mental illness. In mental illness the twofold manner of 'being at home' which is constitutive of human life, being at home in the world and being at home with oneself, is no longer

successfully accomplished. Mental illness does not so much involve the loss of specific abilities as the failure to meet a challenge
with which we are all permanently confronted, that is, of sustaining the equilibrium between our *animalitas* and that in which
we identify our vocation as human beings. When suffering from
mental illness our condition does not simply fall into an animal-
vegetative state; the deforming loss of equilibrium is rather itself
something which peculiarly affects the mind. Structurally this defor-
mation appears, as Bilz has illuminatingly shown,[8] as a potential
virulence which always already belongs to the essential possibilities
of human beings. In my opinion even the complete loss of distance
towards one-self which characterizes certain forms of dementia
must still be seen as a particularly human loss of equilibrium.
Like all loss of equilibrium, 'mental' disturbance too is dialectical,
capable of being restored but also capable of leading finally to
complete destruction through total loss of personality if the
restoration of equilibrium cannot permanently be maintained.
Thus even the dark misfortune of mental illness provides confirmation that a person is not an intelligent animal, but rather a
human being.

Notes

1 Cf. H.-G. Gadamer, *Wahrheit und Methode*, trans. as *Truth and Method*
  (London and New York, 1975); see *Gesammelte Werke* (Tübingen, 1985–),
  vol. 1, pp. 24–35.
2 Since the time of writing, progress in the development of 'artificial intelligence' has fully confirmed the intention of this essay. Cf. also ch. 1 above.
3 F. Nietzsche, *Sämtliche Werke: Kritische Gesamtausgabe*, ed. G. Colli and M.
  Montinari (Berlin, 1967–), p. 40.
4 *Charmides*, 166e ff., and further my 'Vorgestalten der Reflexion', in
  Gesammelte Werke, vol. 6, pp. 116ff.
5 See *Der Nervenarzt*, vol. 35, no. 7 (1964).
6 On Nietzsche cf. my 'Text und Interpretation', in *Gesammelte Werke*, vol. 2,
  no. 24, pp. 330ff.
7 Cf. the much quoted passage from Aristotle's *Politics*, A2, 1253a 13ff. Cf.
  also my essay 'Mensch und Sprache', in *Gesammelte Werke*, vol. 2, no. 11,
  pp. 147ff.
8 See *Der Nervenarzt*, vol. 35 (1964).

4

The Experience of Death

In these reflections I am concerned with more than the mere
change in the representation of death as it has come down to us
through the millennia of human memory, whether in the interpretation provided by religion or in the rituals of everyday life.
I am concerned with a much more radical and specifically contemporary occurrence, that is, with the gradual disappearance of the
representation of death in modern society. This is an event that
clearly demands our consideration. It concerns what I would like
to call a new, second Enlightenment which has now taken hold
of every section of the population and which is entirely based on
the technological control of reality facilitated by the dazzling
achievements of modern natural science and of modern systems
of communication. This second Enlightenment has brought about
a demythologizing of death.

   If one wants to be exact then one should really talk of a
demythologizing of life – and thereby also of death. For that is
the logical order in which the new Enlightenment has unfolded
itself through science. There is something fascinating in the fact
that modern science no longer regards the origin of life in the
universe as a miraculous fact or as the result of an incalculable
play of chance, but is able to identify decisive natural-scientific
causal chains which, through an already largely comprehended

evolutionary process, led to the emergence of life on our planet and all its further developments. On the other hand, we cannot overlook the way in which the industrial revolution and its technological consequences have actually transformed the experience of death in people's lives. It is not only that the funeral procession – prompting everyone to remove their hats before the majesty of death as it drew past – is something that has disappeared from the life of the town. The real depersonalization of death reaches deeper still in the modern hospital. Alongside the loss of any public representation of what takes place, the dying and their relatives are removed from the domestic environment of the family. Death is thereby adapted to the technological business of industrial production. Looking at these changes, we can see that dying has become one of the innumerable processes of production within modern economic life, albeit a negative one. And yet there is perhaps no other experience in human life which so clearly marks the limits placed on that modern control of nature acquired through science and technology. It is precisely these enormous technological advances, with their goal of the artificial preservation of life, which reveal the absolute limit of what we can achieve. The prolongation of life finally becomes a prolongation of death and a fading away of the experience of the self. This process culminates in the gradual disappearance of the experience of death. The anaesthetic drugs developed by modern pharmaceutics can completely sedate the suffering person. The artificial maintenance of the vegetative functions of the organism makes the person into a link in the chain of causal processes. Death itself becomes like an arbitral reward dependent on the decision of the doctor treating the case. At the same time, all this excludes the living from attendance and participation in what is irrevocably taking place. Even the care of the soul which is proffered by the church often fails to gain admittance, and is received neither by the dying person nor by those others who are involved.

At the same time the experience of death occupies a central place in the history of humankind. We could perhaps even say that this experience initiated the process of our becoming human. As far back as human memory extends we can recognize as an undisputed characteristic of human beings that they perform some kind of funeral rites. Already in very early times this was done with a boundless expenditure of ceremony, adornment and art, all devoted to honouring the dead. For the non-specialist it is always a source of astonishment to discover that so many of the splendours of fine art we so admire were in fact votive offerings. In this humankind stands unique among all the other creatures, as unique as in the possession of language. Or perhaps it is something even more original. In any case the evidence of rituals connected with death in early history extends much further back than do the records of human speech.

It is clearly not possible to reconstruct the view of the world which underlay the ancient customs associated with death. However, whatever the religious conceptions of life and death were like which animated the cults surrounding death in the different phases of our early history, there is nevertheless one thing they have in common. They all testify to the fact that humankind neither wanted nor was able to admit that the dead were no longer here, that they had departed, that they finally no longer belonged. This provides unmistakable evidence of a connection between the conscious and self-conscious awareness of our own life and the very ungraspability of death. For every living person there is something incomprehensible in the fact that this human consciousness capable of anticipating the future will one day come to an end. Likewise, for those who witness it, this final coming to an end has something uncanny about it. A beautiful line from the poet Hans Carossa expresses something of this seeming self-evidence of human existence and of its ending. The line runs: 'Wir hören's nicht, wenn Gottes Weise summt, wir hören's erst, wenn sie verstummt' ('We do not hear the murmur of God's song, we hear it only when it ceases').

As regards our enlightened cultural world, it is not inappropriate to speak of an almost systematic repression of death. One need only recall how earlier rites and cultic regulations granted death a ceremonial place in the life of society and how those who were left behind were helped through such rituals to continue their lives and be reincorporated into the community. Something of this still survives today. And yet, for example, the wailing women of ancient cultures, giving dramatic expression to the sorrow of all, are certainly no longer acceptable or even thinkable to modern civilized people.

On the other hand, the repression of death must be conceived as an elementary human reaction to death and one which each human being takes up with respect to their own lives. Thereby the individual is simply responding to the sovereign wisdom of nature concentrated entirely on a single end, to strengthen in every possible way the creature's will to survive when threatened by death. The force of illusion with which the gravely ill or the dying keep hold on their will to live speaks a language which cannot be misunderstood. We must ask ourselves what knowledge of death really means. For there is a deep connection between the knowledge of death, the knowledge of one's own finitude, that is, the certainty that one day one must die, and, on the other hand, the almost imperious demand of not wanting to know, of not wanting to possess this sort of certain knowledge.

In a profound reinterpretation of the oldest mythical traditions, the Greek tragedian Aeschylus, in his drama *Prometheus*, has interpreted the question of death and its meaning for human life. There Prometheus, the friend of man, prides himself that the real service which he performed for mankind was not so much the gift of fire and all the skills bound up with its mastery, but rather that he had taken from us the knowledge of the hour of our death. Before man had been brought by Prometheus this gift of concealment concerning his own death, he must have lived wretchedly and unproductively in caves and created none of those cultural achievements which distinguish mankind above all other living creatures.

The profundity of this account lies in the way the dramatist penetrates behind the traditional legend of the gift of fire and of the awakening of man's practical skills, and thereby reinterprets the ultimate and deepest motivation of the story in terms of this authentic gift. He thus surpasses the cultural pride of the ancient Enlightenment as it was expressed in the formula which Plato puts in the mouth of Protagoras: 'Skill in the arts and fire'

('entechnos sophia sun puri'; *Protagoras*, 321d). It is this motivating reference to death which gives Aeschylus' drama its profundity. The gift consists in the fact that man's very ability to
envisage his own future lends to it such a tangible presence that
he cannot grasp the thought of its actually coming to an end. We
can be said to have a future for as long as we are not aware that
we have no future. The repression of death reflects the will of life.
To this extent knowledge of one's own death is subject to some
remarkable conditions. Thus we can ask ourselves when it is that
a child learns to grasp the fact of death. I am not sure if modern
psychology is able to give any sort of clear answer to this question which would be acceptable to the enlightened society of our
culture. Presumably it is bound up with that inner connection
already described between life and the repression of death that
the knowledge that we ourselves must die remains almost veiled,
even when, as mature adults, this knowledge has become established at the deepest inner level within us. And even then, when
the clearest and most express knowledge of approaching death
makes itself felt and can no longer be concealed, the will to
life and the will towards the future is known to be so strong
in some people that they are not even prepared to complete the
legal requirements of a last testament. Others again treat the
disposal of their estate, as established in their will, almost as a
sort of confirmation of their own life and of their continued
existence.

It can rightly be claimed that the world of modern civilization
eagerly and enthusiastically seeks to bring this tendency to repression which is rooted in life itself to institutional perfection and so
to push the experience of death wholly onto the margins of public
life. Yet it is an astonishing fact that there still remains steadfast
resistance to this cultural tendency. It is not only that religious
ties are sustained in the form of burial services and funeral rites
and often come to life again when there is a bereavement. For
this is even more so in other cultures, especially where religious
tradition has developed richer and more diverse forms, and in
which the force of the modern Enlightenment is only gradually
asserting itself. But even in an age of growing mass atheism such

rituals are still sustained by people who are not believers and who are, in reality, fully secularized. This can be seen in the great festivals of life, the Christian baptism and the Christian marriage, and above all in the funeral ceremonies, the Christian burial and the service of commemoration. Even in atheistic countries Christian or other religious practices are admitted alongside the otherwise political and secular ways of honouring the dead. Even if we must regard this simply as a temporary concession appropriate to a stage of transition, it is none the less very revealing. This is only really valid for the secularized societies of the so-called free world. Everywhere, so to speak, as the obverse side to the repression of death, the consciousness of the living still experiences a fearfulness before the mystery of death, a shuddering before its sacredness, and there is still something uncanny in the silence which accompanies the final parting of someone who was even just now among the living.

Here the genealogical unity of the family in particular seems to sustain a deep-rooted religious vitality. In some cultures, for example in Japan or ancient Rome, the ancestral cult fulfilled a decisive religious function. But in the realm of western Christianity too, the honouring of the dead retained a definite place. This encompassed a whole succession of generations which were preserved in memory and veneration, and in its Christian or other religious guises it formed a sort of counterpart to the normal order of life. In our western world today this may indeed have been completely transformed into rational, this-worldly forms of organization, for example in the contrasting experience of the 'closing down' of graves in our cemeteries. But even in such bureaucratic transactions some knowledge of the unique status of the rite of death is none the less expressed. This can be shown with an example. There is an age-old insight which, beyond all notions of religious transcendence, still reveals its force today. The final parting which death demands from those who are left behind brings about, at the same time, a transformation in the image of the dead person which the living retain in their consciousness and memory. That we should never speak ill of the dead is a prescription that can scarcely be called a prescription.

It is rather an irrepressible need of human nature not only to preserve the character of the dead person, which has been transformed through permanent separation, but to reconstruct it in its productive and positive form. It is changed into an ideal and, as an ideal, becomes itself unchangeable. It is difficult to say what is really taking place in this process whereby, in the final separation from someone, we come to experience their presence in a different way.

By looking at such secularized forms of remembrance it is possible to understand the deep motivations which lie behind religious notions of a beyond and, not least, the need to believe in the immortality of the soul and a reunion after death. The Christian account, which has close parallels in many pagan cults, expresses eloquently how human nature also demands the overcoming of death. What believers experience as an unshakeable certainty and what others experience as perhaps no more than a melancholy yearning is never simply treated as a matter of insignificance which can be lightly brushed aside. It seems as if the repression of death, which belongs to life itself, must be made good again by those who remain among the living in a way which is natural for them. Here both religious faith and purely secular attitudes concur in honouring the majesty of death. The contribution of the scientific Enlightenment reaches an insuperable limit in the mystery of life and of death. Moreover, at this limit a true solidarity of all mankind with one another is expressed in so far as we all recognize and acknowledge this mystery. Whoever lives must accept death. We are all border-crossers at the limit between this world and the beyond.

One would expect that the experience of such a limit, which only religious teachings can claim to transcend or see beyond, would leave philosophical thinking little space for its work of conceptual questioning, grounding and justifying. Above all, however, we must be aware that philosophy cannot even think what is involved for man in the confrontation with death without permanently considering the religious beyond, whether it is the promise of reward or the threat of punishment, as in the Last Judgement. This means, however, for what we call philosophy

that it is only in connection with Greek paganism and the mono-
theism of the Judaic, Christian and Mohammadan religions that
the question of philosophy can be raised at all.

Thus Greek thinking was compelled to ask how the divine can
be thought if the whole force of reality speaks for the inseparable
belonging of life and death and their strict reciprocal exclusive-
ness. As those beings who do not die, as the immortals, the gods
should at the same time represent the highest form of being, that
which is most fully alive. This leads the Greeks to distinguish
within the living being that which does not die and that which
experiences death. They regarded the soul as immortal and, by
giving it the same word, *athanatos*, saw it as participating in the
same state of being as the gods, the immortals. The first Greek
thinker who articulated not only the inner connection between
life and death but that between the immortals and mortals was
Heraclitus in some of his enigmatic fragments. One of them says:
'Immortal mortals, mortal immortals, living their death and dying
their life' (Fragment 62). However this obscure saying is to be
interpreted, it will not be adequately understood unless *psyche*, the
soul, is adequately grasped as something in which mutually antagonistic moments are entwined.

This train of thought is pursued in Plato's *Phaedo*, which
presents the dialogue of the condemned Socrates with his friends
on the day at the end of which he was to drink from the poisoned
cup. The religious composure with which Socrates here examines
and rejects every argument which would deny the immortality of
the soul is the strongest encouragement which we can find in the
ancient world for that child in us who cannot be fully consoled
by any argument. The dying Socrates becomes exemplary for all
who come after him. I need recall only the Stoic sage and his im-
perturbability in the face of death, whereby he demonstrates his
own freedom. The trial of steadfast free decision was demanded
even for the act of suicide, which was not forbidden for the
Stoics. For their religion permitted death, but only through pro-
longed fasting or through gradual bleeding to death in full consciousness of what was taking place. We are familiar, too, with
the example of the Epicureans. They combated the fear of death

through argument and at the same time brought the art of life to its highest perfection. Lessing, equally as a humanist and as a child of the modern Enlightenment, emphasized in a well-known treatise that the ancients thought of death and represented it as the brother of sleep rather than as the fearful skeleton of the Christian Middle Ages.

But today we all live under the conditions of the modern Enlightenment. Access to a transfiguring world of consolation such as Lessing describes remains, in the last analysis, closed to us. It constitutes the harshness and severity of the modern Enlightenment that it is the result of a science which itself developed out of the Christian transformation of pagan antiquity. The transcendence of God imposed on human knowledge the task of learning about humankind itself and so, finally, transformed the task of acquiring knowledge as such. A new attitude to quantification and a new ideal of rational construction founded a new empire. It is governed by the ideal of mastery through knowledge, and by means of scientific investigation it permanently extends the limits of what can be controlled. But if it is true that even this scientific Enlightenment, like that of the ancient world, finds its limit in the ungraspability of death, then it remains true that the horizon of questioning within which thought can approach the enigma of death at all is still circumscribed by doctrines of salvation. For us, this is the doctrine of Christianity in all its diversity of churches and sects. To reflective thinking it must seem as ungraspable as it is illuminating that the true overcoming of death cannot lie in anything but the resurrection of the dead. For those who believe, this is the greatest certainty, while for those who do not it remains something ungraspable, but no more ungraspable than death itself.

5

Bodily Experience and the Limits of Objectification

Today I want to present what is still a very modest attempt to reflect on the theme of the living body, embodiment and objectification. I want to make us explicitly aware of what everyone fundamentally already knows, that modern science and its ideal of objectification demands of all of us a violent estrangement from ourselves, irrespective of whether we are doctors, patients or simply responsible and concerned citizens.

This is all the more necessary since the philosophical tradition to which I too belong, both as a student of the Marburg School and as a phenomenologist and student of Husserl and Heidegger, has done little to illuminate the theme of the body and embodiment and its peculiar obscurity. It is no accident that Heidegger himself was forced to admit that he had not reflected on the theme of the body or concentrated his intellectual powers on it to the same extent as he had on so many other essential themes of human existence. Nor, I think, is it an accident that Edmund Husserl, with his astonishing phenomenological-analytical talent, saw the description of the sphere of individuality and everything connected with the experience of the body and the way it is phenomenologically 'given' – the whole wealth of kinaesthetic phenomena in which the body is felt and experienced – as indeed an essential task but none the less as one which takes us to the very limits of the possible.

If we consider these facts, we are confronted with a fundamental question. We must ask whether the present world situation does not present us with specifically human responsibilities, and whether modern science with its ethos of achievement, which has brought these responsibilities to a critical point, is not forcing western culture towards a critical self-examination? This is something we need to recognize. This is why I have explicitly pointed out the significance of the fact that we are moving into a global civilization in which our perfected technical achievements are encountering new and different traditions of cultural life. This may even provide fresh impetus for the task of addressing our human responsibilities.

The phrase 'the body and embodiment', like 'the living body and life', sounds almost like a play on words and thus acquires for us an almost mysterious presence. It vividly presents the absolute inseparability of the living body and life itself. We should perhaps even ask ourselves whether questions concerning the existence of the soul, indeed any talk of the soul at all, could ever arise if we did not experience the body both as something living and as something subject to decay. Perhaps, even for us today, Aristotle was right when he said that the soul is nothing more than the living character of the body, the form of fulfilled self-realization which he called *entelecheia*.

On the other hand, we can take up an external view on the world and observe, among all its various phenomena, our own bodily experience. Through its methodological procedures modern science has succeeded in objectifying this experience. This is something science cannot avoid doing and we cannot ignore its consequences for praxis. This does not mean, however, that we are not able to identify limits as to what can be known in this way and that this, in turn, cannot awaken a hermeneutic awareness concerning the limits of objectification in general. We would then have to ask: what is the relationship between science and bodily experience? How does the one arise out of the other? Can science be connected once again with our own lived experience, or must the experience of one's own individuality be lost irrevocably in the context of modern data banks and new technology? This is the question which I want to address in these reflections. It is one which concerns the fate of our western civilization as a whole. For who knows if or how the increasing perfection of our instrumentally orientated thought can be brought into a new and fruitful interaction with the humane values of other cultures and with our own partially buried tradition? The first question which confronts us if we want to try to resolve the enigma concerning our own embodiment is why this phenomenon is so intractable and resistant to thematization. It is clear that mankind has always reflected on the mystery of the living body. For there has always been illness. Every culture has had its practitioners of medicine or those considered wise enough to come to the aid of the sick, even if they did so without possessing a corresponding scientific expertise. How, then, was the practice of healing integrated within the totality of the social world and what is the prospect for this today?

What does it mean to become aware of the body as the body and to treat it as such? What is this tiny, fragile and ephemeral thing that sustains our life in the vast totality of the world? What is our place in the totality of things? In raising such questions it will immediately become clear to everyone that we are touching on a theme of fundamental significance. The body and its distinction from something like the soul, whether this is understood in a religious or some other sense, is an inescapable topos of thought. How is the fact of our embodiment related to the mysterious phenomenon of reflective consciousness, which is capable of thinking out beyond all temporal and corporeal constraints and even of losing itself in the infinite? How is this related to our responsibility as human beings, as thinking natural beings, and how can we successfully reconnect our instrumental reason, especially in light of the vast scale of its modern development, with the totality of our being-in-the-world in a fruitful and productive way? How are we to approach this task at all?

In my 'Apologia for the Art of Healing' (chapter 2) and

discussion of other related themes, I began from the Greek experience of the world. It would certainly seem natural to turn to the resources of our western tradition in order to develop critical reflections concerning the future. Something which has long guided me in my reflections about such things is a famous passage in Plato's *Phaedrus*. This concerns the recognition that, as certain famous Greek physicians had observed, the body cannot be treated without at the same time treating the soul. It is further suggested that perhaps even this is not enough, that it is impossible to treat the body without possessing knowledge concerning the whole of being. In Greek the whole of being is *hole ousia*. Anyone knowing this phrase in Greek will also hear, alongside the expression 'the whole of being', the suggestion of 'hale and healthy being'. The being whole of the whole and the being healthy of the whole, the healthiness of well-being, seem to be most intimately related. In German when one is unwell one says 'Es fehlt mir etwas' – literally, I am lacking in something.

What can we learn from these etymological considerations? We need to recognize that it is only through a disturbance of the whole that a genuine consciousness of the problem and a genuine concentration of thought upon it can arise. I know only too well how illness can make us insistently aware of our bodily nature by creating a disturbance in something which normally, in its very freedom from disturbance, almost completely escapes our attention. Here it is a matter of the methodological primacy of illness over health. But of course it is the state of being healthy which possesses ontological primacy, that natural condition of life which we term well-being, in so far as we register it at all. But what is well-being if it is not precisely this condition of not noticing, of being unhindered, of being ready for and open to everything?

Wolfgang Blankenburg once used the expression 'it is there'. Through Heidegger we have all learnt that this sense of 'it is there' does not have the thing-like character of an object. It is for this reason, of course, that Blankenburg used it to characterize our experience of the body. The decisive point is that in this 'it is there', in our being given over to the world, in our state of openedness and openness, in our spiritual receptivity for everything, whatever it may be, we are also there ourselves. For this the Greeks possessed – and I must apologize for constantly using such beautiful Greek words – the term *nous*. This word originally referred to the scenting of the air by a wild beast when it sensed nothing more than 'there is something there'. But the term can only properly be applied to human beings, since we possess this awesome capacity to give ourselves over to something completely and to allow what is other to be entirely 'there' in its own right. This perspective allows my proper theme, sickness and embodiment, to become accessible in a particular way.

In German a doctor will begin by asking 'Na, wo fehlt's denn?', or 'what's the matter with you then?', literally, 'what are you lacking?' Or we ourselves may ask 'Was fehlt mir eigentlich?', literally, 'what am I lacking?' This is a question which we as patients can address to a doctor who is about to examine us or give us advice. Is it not an extraordinary thing that the lack of something, although we do not know precisely what it is that is lacking, can reveal the miraculous existence of health? It is only now, in its absence, that I notice what was previously there, or, more precisely, not *what* was previously there but *that* it was there. This is what one calls well-being. We also say 'I am fine.' Here we encounter wakefulness and being-in-the-world as authentic presence. Here presence does not refer to that mysterious aspect of time in the narrow sense of a series of temporal points which are enumerated in their momentary being. Rather, presence refers here to something which fully occupies a kind of space. Thus we say of great actors that they have presence. For such an actor simply being on the stage suffices, while the others must constantly exert themselves. Or, with outstanding statesmen, we notice their stature and presence when they enter a room. This is a kind of presence in which our authentic existence, so to speak, realizes its telos, its perfected form. The word *entelecheia* is the marvellous expression which Aristotle fashioned to express this. He thereby created a word which in itself, as it were, articulates the full completion and realization of a living being. But what is it then that rises up against this, what is the disturbance which estranges us from everything around us when something is felt to be 'lacking', when we feel ourselves to be unwell?

Rainer Maria Rilke died sixty years ago from a grave and incurable blood disease in a Swiss hospital. In the very last verses he wrote, in the face of the searing pain which was consuming him, he expressed how the pain alienated him from himself. He wrote: 'Oh life, life, remaining always outside.' So powerfully does pain cause us to withdraw from all external experience of the world and turn us back upon ourselves. Such experience at the point of extremity contains a universal truth, one which has not merely been impressed on us by the Christian religion and the passion story which has accompanied us since childhood. Every culture knows something of the profound inwardization involved in suffering and the endurance of pain. Here we face the real difficulty at the heart of our theme. On the one hand, there is the remarkable protected state in which we feel ourselves safely enfolded so that we are able, lightly and effortlessly, to embrace our desire for active participation in life. But on the other hand, we know the oppressive weight of things which bear down on us, dragging us downwards towards those dark demons which our medical colleagues describe in terms of hypochondria and depression. We have all experienced something of this. Just think what is at play between these extremes of soaring confidence and profound depression! What specifically human contribution can we make to these problems when, as doctors, we are in possession of an increasing capacity for instrumental control over the body?

I ask myself whether the Greeks did not perhaps possess a broader framework within which to meet such a challenge than we do. We find evidence for this in that section of the *Phaedrus* which speaks of the well-being of the body, the well-being of the soul and the well-being of the whole in a single context. Again in Plato's great utopia of the *Republic* the true part of the citizen in the ideal state is described in terms of health, as a harmony in which everything is in accord, in which even the fateful problem of governing and being governed is resolved through reciprocal agreement and mutual interaction. The whole mystery of *harmonia*, this sounding together in agreement of differing voices, can be heard in our own language when we talk of the concordance of dissonances. Among the fragments of Heraclitus we find this profound observation: 'The concealed harmony is mightier than the revealed.' Did Heraclitus here have in mind the enigma of health? In thinking about these questions I have attempted to take my bearings from, among other things, the problem of pain. We notice how pain and the suffering it inflicts change in character when they are no longer accompanied by the certainty or the expectation that it can be eliminated. This is something we know from contemporary medicine with its virtuosic capacity to 'eliminate' pain, the source of the pain, the symptom and sometimes even more than this. By means of its capacity to remove pain in this way modern medicine changed the role and importance within human life of certain illnesses which can be so quickly dealt with today. One simply takes something for it and then it is gone. Viktor von Weizsäcker, with whom I often had the opportunity of speaking before his own ill-health prevailed, always used to ask: what does illness tell the one who is ill? Not so much, what does it tell the doctor, but rather, what does it tell the patient? Can learning to ask such a question of oneself perhaps even contribute to helping the one who is ill?

In the case of transient illnesses and 'eliminable' pain we have learnt to regard them as no longer important. Consequently modern medicine has principally seen itself confronted by chronic illnesses and the different challenges they present. For here it is a question of tending the ill, which also requires attending to their mental and emotional well-being. But what does this new status of chronic illnesses within modern medicine mean? Clearly one must learn to accept such illness and attempt to live with it as far as the illness in question will allow. What conclusion can be drawn from this for that extremity of illness which finds such powerful expression in Rilke's poem? Illness of this kind is not to be confused with all the other illnesses we have endured in our lives and from which we have expected to recover. Should we simply learn to live with illness, even with chronic illness, where life itself is at stake?

At the limits of this question the lay person enters a mysterious and remote terrain, that realm of profound emotional disturbance and mental illness which psychiatrists must work with. What is this condition which does not really belong among the organic illnesses and which we are scarcely able to describe in terms of the bodily organism? Here it is not a question of the resistance still shown by the body which has fallen victim to illness. There is no 'it hurts' or 'there is something wrong here'. All of that may be described as a disturbance in our state of well-being. In the case of well-being is enough to be able to say that one feels well, and to mean by that the ability to be completely involved in something else, in whatever else it is that one wants to do. But here we are speaking of a completely different type of disturbance, something that belongs to a different and mysterious world. Admittedly, even this domain has to a certain extent become accessible to us through the sophisticated development of new medical techniques. I am thinking, for example, of the world of modern psychiatric drugs. But I cannot separate this development from the general instrumentalization of the living body which also occurs in the world of modern agriculture, in the economy and in industrial research. What does it signify that such instrumentalization now defines what we are and what we are capable of achieving? Does this not also open up a new threat to human life? Is there not a terrifying challenge involved in the fact that through psychiatric drugs doctors are able not only to eliminate and deaden various organic disturbances, but also to take away from a person their own deepest distress and confusion? Here we cannot really speak of a simple 'taking away' as if we were in total control. It seems to me of great importance that this radical form of disturbance which we do not even properly term an illness – as when we talk, for example, of someone being mentally 'disturbed' – requires us to recognize the central role played by speech and dialogue. And by this I do not simply mean therapeutic dialogue, as it has been developed by psychoanalysis in the strict sense. Rather, I mean that in all medical treatment the patient needs to receive guidance, and here the discussion and shared dialogue between doctor and patient plays a decisive role. What we can learn from this conception of the full realization of the doctor–patient relationship as it ought to prevail is that for all these forms of disturbance it is less a case of 'taking something away' than of assisting in the process of adaptation and reentry into the cycle of human, social, professional and family life. And this is something which transpires in the shared medium of communication between human beings. The extreme case of mental disturbance, where we attempt to help someone to rediscover their own internal balance and equilibrium, strikes me as prototypical for the general experience of disturbance and the task of readaptation with which humankind has always been confronted, and with which it always will be confronted.

Here lies my own deepest hope, or perhaps I should say, dream: that from the shared inheritance which is gradually being built up for us from all the different human cultures across the globe we might eventually learn how to recognize our needs and address our difficulties through becoming explicitly conscious of them. The life of the body always seems to me to be something which is experienced as a constant movement between the loss of equilibrium and the search for a new point of stability. What a remarkable thing it is that a slight pitch in balance counts as nothing, that we can tilt almost until falling and then swing back into equilibrium. Yet, on the other hand, whenever we go beyond this point of balance, we fall into irreversible misfortune. This seems to me to be the fundamental model for our bodily, and not merely bodily, existence as human beings.

We can learn a great deal from the experience of our own embodied nature which is suggested by this model. It reveals the rhythm of sleeping and waking, the rhythm of illness and recovery, and finally, at the end, the transition into nothingness, the expiring movement of life itself. These are temporal structures which modulate the entire course of our lives. They confirm what was said by the Greek physician Alkmaion, that human beings cannot connect the end again with the beginning, and for this reason must die. Alkmaion clearly and appropriately describes the rhythm of our living being from the perspective of our end, our ultimate or 'limit situation'. The rhythmic order of what we call our vegetative life, lived by us all, can never be replaced completely by an 'instrumentalized' relation to the body, any more than death can ever be eliminated. 'Death in Hollywood' has shown

us this in an unforgettable way. Although there is a great deal
that we can hide and repress, fabricate and replace, even a doctor who is able to help patients survive critical phases of their
organic life through the extraordinary means of automated
and mechanical substitutes for functioning organs is still, eventually, forced to recognize the patient as an individual human being.
This takes place when, finally, the doctor is confronted with the
momentous decision as to when the instrumental preservation
of the patient's merely vegetative existence can, or ought to be,
withdrawn. From this 'limit situation', and here I use again a
significant term which Karl Jaspers introduced, we can learn
something concerning the many different limits which are placed
on us. We must ask ourselves what science and its facility for
objectification ought to mean for us. What can intervention, our
own actions, our dependency on the help of others, and our perhaps even greater dependency on helping ourselves, contribute
towards bringing the achievements of modern society, with all of
its automated, bureaucratized and technologized apparatus, back
into the service of that fundamental rhythm which sustains the
proper order of bodily life?

Today we see and hear a great deal about an emergent ecological
consciousness. This is perhaps one of the first hopeful signs in
our critical world situation. I find it remarkable that here we use
a word which hardly plays any role in our everyday lives any
longer. The Greek word *oikos* meant the domestic house and in
this connection we also speak of the 'household'. One learns to
keep house with the means, energy and time that are available.
The Greek word, however, means something more than this. For
it includes not only the ability to manage by one's self, but also
the ability to manage along with other people. One form of help
which each of us can provide for ourselves, it seems to me, is to
learn properly how to integrate this reliance on one another·into
our own lived existence. This is rather analogous to the way we
are able on occasion to register, as it were, something of the self-
sustaining rhythm of our own bodily life. Without paying explicit
attention to its course and gentle fluctuations, we succeed none
the less, through unconscious reaction, in sustaining this rhythm

by instinctive relaxation and the ability to rediscover the easy enjoyment of our own life and activity.

We need to see then what the problems we have addressed concerning the living body, its resistance to thematization and its tendency to become perspicuous only sporadically by virtue of some disturbance, can teach us about how we are to deal with our whole cultural apparatus and all its various instrumental possibilities. This requires the other abilities involved in keeping house which are, perhaps, more important than those of thrift and which will always prove necessary to a well-kept household. These not only encompass myself and my own activities but also include the house as a whole. The house is what is held in common, it is both the familiar practices and the dwelling place where people are at home together. This is not really something we need to learn about all over again. It is something we all know, but we have forgotten its paradigmatic importance and to that extent need to remember it once more.

I would not like to fall under the suspicion that these reflections merely betray the unchecked desire of a very old man to develop perspectives on the future from out of our present darkness. On the contrary, I still believe that I am right to claim that we must rigorously deny the possibility that human life can be lived without a future. For, as I see it, it is a distinctively human fact that we must always keep the future open and with it new possibilities. If I start out from this fundamental conviction then I am sure that there is a great deal, in small things as well as in large, that we ought gradually to develop more practice in doing. Perhaps in the long term even for our society, driven as it is by the notion of progress, we can generate once again a sense of good housekeeping, both for oneself and for others, and succeed in raising a sense of responsibility which goes beyond ourselves into a self-evident and conscious value. It is not so impossible that fear, want and need will eventually bring us to reason. This can also take place across the planet as a whole. The so-called underdeveloped countries cannot at present believe that there are ecological problems for humankind that might concern them. They consider our protective measures merely those of the *beati possidentes*. It is true that we cannot see paths and solutions in advance, and yet we must ask ourselves if there will not always remain new possibilities. We encounter, for example, the loss of personhood. This happens within medical science when the individual patient is objectified in terms of a mere multiplicity of data. In a clinical investigation all the information about a person is treated as if it could be adequately collated on a card index. If this is done correctly, then the relevant data will all uniquely apply to the person involved. But the question is whether the unique value of the individual is properly recognized in this process.

Clearly this is not merely true for the situation of patients within the institution of the clinic. In the vast technical structure of our civilization we are all patients. Our personal existence is clearly something which is everywhere denied and yet it is also something which is always involved in the attempt to regain that balance which we need for ourselves, for our lived environment and for the feeling of being at home in the world. It extends far beyond the sphere of medical responsibility and includes the integration of individuals into their family, social and professional lives. This does not seem to me to be an abstract task, but rather something concrete which permanently confronts us. The challenge is the continual one of sustaining our own internal balance within a larger social whole which requires both cooperation and participation. It seems to me that there are many situations in which we are in a position not only to identify problems which restrict us but also to discover new possibilities for a more humane arrangement of things as they have been developed in our instrumentalized social organization. This is something we occasionally realize through the encounter with another human being. For example, sometimes, hearing a politician speak, we find it impossible to escape the pull of their ideas and projects because we feel ourselves and our concerns to have been understood.

However, our social existence is so organized and so constrained that such encounters are difficult and rarely take place. I do not want to start enumerating here all the possibilities for a more humane treatment of human beings. With my last remarks I would like to refer to certain issues raised in my own thinking and in what I have called hermeneutic experience. Here it is a question of recognizing and actualizing something which I consider to be a presupposition of our being human, namely that the other may not only have a right but may actually be right, may understand something better than we do. There is a marvellous essay by Kierkegaard called 'On what is edifying in the thought that we are always wrong in the face of God'. There is a great consolation in this because so often we are indeed in the wrong and because it is so difficult to admit to it. We have, as it were, to learn to recognize in our errors and presumptions that these are in fact only limited realizations of real superiority and unavoidable inferiority with respect to knowledge. Thus in my opinion we should extend our understanding of the relationship which obtains between doctor and patient and which underlies the paradox of the non-objectifiability of the living body to all our experience of limits and conditions. This relationship is in no way an exceptional one. Today I see the problem of modern instrumental reason more in terms of its application to things with which we are all concerned, whether it is as teacher or as family member, in the school or in some other institution of public life. We cannot and should not lead young people to believe that they will inherit a future of satisfying comfort and increasing ease. Rather, we should convey to them a pleasure in collective responsibility and in a genuinely shared existence both with and for one another. This is something which is missing both in our society and indeed in many others as well. Young people in particular are well aware of this. And here we are reminded of an ancient saying: youth is in the right.

6

Between Nature and Art

It is difficult in a short space of time to say something self-contained about a man such as Viktor von Weizsäcker and his achievements, about the problems on which he worked and on which we must continue to work. Perhaps you will allow my contribution today to be understood as a continuation of the ongoing discussion with Viktor von Weizsäcker which I took up with him on the occasions when we met. As a lay person in the domain of medical science and the art of medicine I was not, of course, in a position to participate productively in questions concerning strictly medical problems. However, I have continued to occupy myself with the theme of the *Gestaltkreis* as well as the figure of this brooding Schwabian thinker who was capable of concealing his thoughts in an almost cryptic way.

For me Weizsäcker's *Gestaltkreis* finally became more like a symbolic idea, an invitation to participate in a shared reflection on certain problems, something which I hoped to be able to do again when I returned to Heidelberg in 1949 and could renew my contact with Viktor von Weizsäcker. Sadly, we were no longer able to carry on these conversations because of his ill-health. Today, then, in place of a productive contribution of my own, I would like to discuss some of those questions which I had wanted to ask him. The things I have been most concerned with, and which still concern me, are certainly not restricted to the special competence of doctors and their particular domain of reflective experience. In putting these questions forward here under the title 'Between Nature and Art' I am not proposing to make a contribution to what, in our normal use of language, is generally understood by 'art'. Rather, I am referring to that totality of skills and abilities which is known to us all and which can be seen as the special and dangerous gift which has been bequeathed to mankind. I mean 'art' here in the sense of the ancients, as *techne*, that knowledge and knowing ability which Greek antiquity first developed in the direction of those skills and sciences which today embrace the world. This was the ultimate theme, as it were, which I hoped to embark on in the discussions with Viktor von Weizsäcker which were not destined to take place.

It is certainly not necessary to belong to western civilization or to have been brought up within its particular frame of conceptual thought in order to be clearly aware of the peculiar position humankind occupies within the whole of that nature which both surrounds and supports us. The natural cycle of things which takes place all around us was looked on as something exemplary both in the earliest forms of human thought and in our own western cultural tradition. This latter, for good reason, is also termed a *Kulturkreis*, or cultural sphere. We find this in Plato, for example, when he undertook to describe all the different visions of the world which he had either witnessed or was bold enough to entertain. He sought to reveal the interweaving connections which bind the spheres of the soul, the city state and the universe as a whole. This awareness must be regarded as a form of higher wisdom when compared to the hubris which inspires our own ever-expanding technical capacities and abilities. None the less, this capacity for technical mastery represents something distinctively human, and ultimately it is this which has given rise to the critical situation in which the human race finds itself on the planet today. We have developed our knowledge and technical abilities to such a pitch that they now represent a fundamental, all-embracing attitude towards nature and the human world.

Moreover, we continue to promote their further development without measure. This is the crisis in which we find ourselves and we can only hope that, like the critical point of an illness, this will lead us towards a new equilibrium in the respective spheres of the body, the soul and the harmony of the world as a whole. What Viktor von Weizsäcker used to call the *Gestaltkreis*, this ongoing interplay between perception and movement, was also recognized in the deepest wisdom of the Greeks. They held *krinein*, the ability to discriminate, and *kinein*, the power of movement, to be the specific characteristics which distinguish living creatures within the totality of nature. We too are such living creatures. But we are creatures who have been endowed by nature itself with the capacity to take up a bold and possibly perilous distance in relation to our own natural being. By virtue of this endowment we are 'exposed' in a special way. We are, in particular, exposed to an awareness of our own future. For a human being is the creature who can think the future and who seeks to know how things will be in advance. But this distinguishing characteristic of human beings is also what makes them dangerous even to themselves.

It would be presumptuous to evaluate the achievements of an individual, or even of a generation or a particular stage in our historical development, without recognizing the greatness of the achievement of western civilization as a whole. A mantle of civilization, beneath which other developed and developing countries are almost hidden from view, arose in Europe and today covers the entire world. People's 'exposed' condition, though true of all humankind, has been intensified in western civilization to the point of endangering us all. We should consider it a universal responsibility of human beings to learn to turn this capacity for directing our attention away from ourselves – this permanent orientation towards new possibilities, towards the unknown, towards new ventures – back in the direction of the vast, balance-sustaining rhythm of the natural order. This is something which is revealed to us in the course of each and every day. The mystery of sleep seems to me to be one of those fundamental experiences in which our human self-understanding reveals itself both as something continuous with nature and yet as something which constantly strives towards establishing the new. Every morning of every day each of us experiences the promise and the risk involved in a new day and a new morrow. It is precisely here, in the movement between sleep and waking, between relaxation and exertion, that we encounter the peculiar constitution of human beings, their capacity to abandon themselves to the pursuit of the most daring goals while retaining their own self-identity. This is something which we find belongs to our fundamental constitution. Doctors who have thought about such matters will, accordingly, recognize that the most fundamental challenge which faces them is not simply to aid the recovery of the person who is sick. Rather, they are confronted with the challenge of restoring to patients their own sense of self-identity by enabling them to return to and take up again their own particular way of life and to exercise their own particular abilities.

It does not seem to me to be a mere accident that Viktor von Weizsäcker decided to continue his career as a doctor even though he was highly gifted in many different fields. As a physiologist in the school of von Kries he could have pursued a great academic career, and as a tenacious and reflective thinker with an openness and sensitivity to the mystery of life he could also have dedicated himself completely to the pursuit of philosophy. However, in each and every important decision in his life he decided ultimately to carry on working with those who are ill, and herein we see a confirmation of his human and personal qualities. It was in the face of illness that he sought to discover the great enigma of health, and it was here that he sought to provide what assistance he could.

During the war I once experienced this for myself, as a professor at the University of Leipzig, when the chair of psychology fell vacant. The Leipzig school of experimental psychology had previously occupied a leading position throughout the entire world. The Psychological Institute of Wilhelm Wundt was the very first to be founded. In 1944, with the agreement of the faculty, I invited Viktor von Weizsäcker to take up the post as successor to the psychologist Lersch who had been called to Munich. I knew, I think, what I was doing. I also understood why Herr von Weizsäcker responded to this attempt to bring him there as if to a very strong temptation. Finally, however, he decided to give up all such plans and to return to Heidelberg from Breslau. The attraction the position must have held for him was clearly the same as that which made us so want to give it to him. We would have succeeded in recalling a scientist back into general psychology, and thus at the same time back into philosophy, disciplines in great need of new forms and powers of reflection. At that time psychology had long since progressed beyond its origins in empirical physiology and the contemporary problems of experimental empirical psychology. In the effort to open up new areas of human psychological experience to scientific analysis it had degenerated into a diffuse range of vague typological and pragmatic studies. This task of leading the discipline of psychology back towards the primary phenomena of the *condition humaine* seemed to us one which was worthy of such a highly accomplished scientist and open-minded thinker. And we all shared the conviction that such a task really only manifests itself fully in the context of pain, illness, and the human experience of lack which this involves. The mystery of illness bears witness to the great miracle of health, that it allows us to live in the happiness of forgetting, in a state of well-being, of lightness and ease. At that time we were motivated by the idea that a doctor who possessed the fundamental natural-scientific training of an experimental researcher and yet was also able to direct his reflections across the entire spectrum of human experience could collaborate with our own work in a collective project. Of course, in the late stages of the war this was an illusion. But living in a country which was guilty of plunging itself into ruin and which was caught in a process of degeneration, we needed to believe in new possibilities for the future and were capable of harbouring such illusions.

Herr von Weizsäcker saw with great clarity that ultimately it was more important for him to return to Heidelberg and his medical practice than it was to take part in our work in Leipzig which was leading into unknown theoretical territory. I include this biographical information simply to explain why it was that I held discussions with Herr von Weizsäcker both before his return to Heidelberg, and then subsequently when I too decided to go there. I hoped to discuss with him the mystery of the *Kreis*, the mystery of this self-sustaining infinite process which is revealed in organic life and which, as every reader of Plato knows, is the subject of an unforgettable passage of the *Phaedrus*. Here Socrates says to his young companion that we cannot know anything about the human soul, or even anything about the human body, without already knowing something of the whole, the *holon* of nature. For those who know Greek this word has a special ring. It is not simply equivalent to our German expression *das Ganze*, meaning the whole or the entirety. For *holon* is also that which is intact or undamaged, that which is sound and healthy. It is that process which, by virtue of its own self-contained and self-producing living power, finds its place within the totality of nature. Doctors must be fully aware of this when they are dealing with all the different tasks which confront them. We must remember how deeply Viktor von Weizsäcker thought about these questions when he attempted to grasp the 'untruth' of illness. He asked what it is that is hidden from us, what remains concealed, when our state of physical health falls into division with itself. Do we not have something to learn from what happens when we fall ill, from that condition we find ourselves in before we return to the state of well-being, with all the incredible and inconceivable ease that such a return brings with it?

The example which Plato gives can help us here. Plato says, or rather, lets Socrates say, that perhaps the physician must know not only the nature of the soul but the nature of the 'whole' to be able really to treat the patient's experience of lack, of illness and pain.

Over thousands of years of experience we have been told, and we know, how this task has developed into an 'art' of great difficulty. This difficulty has only been increased by the new obligations and achievements which result from our increasingly specialized knowledge and abilities. The process of historical development has not only placed the roles of patient and doctor ever more under the law of the division of labour, but has done the same with the lives of us all. This has reduced our own contribution to that of a mere function within a whole which is no longer easily surveyable. In this context the doctor's profession possesses in a certain sense a symbolic value. For the task which confronts the doctor is not one of 'making' something but rather one of providing help, of enabling patients to recover their health and to return to their everyday lives. Doctors can never completely entertain the illusion that health is something they simply 'make' or which they can fully control. They know that it is not themselves or their abilities but rather nature which they help to victory. It is this which characterizes the unique position of medicine within human science as a whole. It is true that all our various capacities and all our claims to knowledge are conditioned, that our power to 'make' things is always limited by the bounds set by nature. But medicine is the only science which, ultimately, does not make or produce anything. Rather, it is one which must participate in the wonderful capacity of life to renew itself, to set itself aright. The real task which confronts the doctor is that of assisting in this process of restoration or recovery. Recovery here does not only mean a return to the harmony of waking and sleeping, of metabolic change, of respiration and all the other vital functions involved in life which someone who has been sick must learn to coordinate once again. It also means meeting the challenge of finding a way back from the condition of social disruption which illness entails and of taking up again one's work or occupation, the sphere in which we actually live our lives. This is something we all know. Already in the Old Testament, in the Book of Genesis, the vocation of human labour is recognized not merely as a curse of eternal toil but also, in a certain sense, as a wise endowment given to humankind. And herein lies our real task: to recognize our unique position between nature and art, to recognize that we are both natural creatures and yet in possession of special abilities. This is something we can come to understand by considering the role doctors play and the special character their abilities possess. It is precisely the work of doctors and their 'achievements' that can make us aware of the limits placed on our human technical skills. Our proper task is to learn to recognize and to accept these limits.

This is the first and foremost thing which, even from out of what we have called the untruth of illness, is capable of finally leading truth to victory. It is the truth that is concealed in all illness and in every threat to life and well-being. What this truth reveals is the unshakeable will to life, the inviolable forces of hope and vitality which we all possess as our most natural endowment. It can teach us to recognize that which is given, that which limits us and causes us pain. To learn to accept illness for what it is – this is perhaps one of the great changes brought about in our modern civilization by the progress of medicine. This presents us with new challenges. It is surely not without significance that today doctors seem to be able almost to conjure away so many illnesses, so that for the patient they simply disappear without anything having been learnt from them. Significantly, it is now the chronic illnesses which stand at the forefront of medical interest, precisely because they cannot simply be 'taken away'. In fact the most chronic of all illnesses is the path which leads us towards death. To learn to accept this is the highest task of humankind.

When I call to mind the figure of Viktor von Weizsäcker as I remember him, I always connect him with what we have said here about the task of being human. There was something enigmatic about him. He possessed a pensive and brooding mind, but then suddenly he would light up and the brilliant observational power of a great doctor would combine with his humanity and openness towards others. This is how I remember him, and not only as a doctor who could help us to reestablish that equilibrium which is granted to us by nature. He was also able, like every great doctor, to teach us to accept our own limits and, himself aware of the ultimate task of humanity, he was able to accept his own ultimate limits. For this reason I would like to close with a few lines from a poem. I do so, not so much to compensate for any possible misunderstandings that may have arisen from my choice of the title 'Art and Nature', but rather because I think it bears valid testimony to what I have said here.

It is a poem by Ernst Meister, an early student of mine who, shortly before his death, was awarded the Georg Büchner prize. The poem reads:

> Immer noch
> laß ich mich glauben
> es gäbe
> ein Recht des Gewölbes,
> die krumme Wahrheit
> des Raumes.
> Vom Auge gebogen,
> Unendlichkeit,
> himmlisch,
> sie biegt das Eisen,
> den Willen,
> sterblich,
> ein Gott zu sein.

(I still allow myself to believe that there exists an order in the vault of the heavens, in the arched truth of space. Though bent by the human eye this heavenly infinity itself bends iron, bends the will, though mortal yet to be a god.)

7

Philosophy and Practical Medicine

I come here as a lay person into a group with which I have long felt myself to be connected. My friendship with Viktor von Weizsäcker goes back to the 1930s and since then I have kept a close relationship with many of his colleagues and students in Heidelberg. But, sadly, one does not always gain as much as one might wish from such close proximity. Perhaps I may be allowed to recall the words of Socrates, who was invited to a celebration in honour of one of the great tragedians, Agathon.[1] Finding himself seated between Agathon and the famous comic dramatist Aristophanes, Socrates remarked: 'It would be a fine thing if wisdom were like water which can flow from one vessel into another along a piece of worsted. Then I would be able to learn a great deal from those sitting next to me' (*Symposium*, 175d). However, as Socrates confirms, this is unfortunately not the case, and I still remain unclear about many things despite my long-standing connection with this group. I even find the title which has been announced somewhat troubling. What is the specifically 'philosophical' dimension which is at stake here? This is something I have thought about again and again in the hope of discovering a plausible answer. How should I begin to understand what has been asked of me here? Clearly it belongs to the essence of philosophy in contrast to the other sciences that it raises questions which we cannot eliminate even if we do not know how to answer them. In this sense the question concerning the nature of philosophy is itself a philosophical question to which we have no answer. Whatever philosophy is, it must be seen as a natural propensity within us all rather than as some sort of professional skill or ability. I ask of you, then, that my contribution today be understood not as that of a specialist who has answers to all the questions, but rather as that of one who is simply putting forward his own reflections alongside everyone else's.

Even in the age of science there still exists one indisputable domain which remains common to us all. I refer to language, to that ongoing dialogue we all sustain with one another. In language, experience and knowledge become sedimented and speak directly to us through the words themselves. I would like to make my contribution to the theme which stands before us for discussion today by starting out from some reflections about specific words.

The second half of our title, 'practical medicine', has also given me food for thought. It is often remarked how important the theme of 'general medicine' has become for us. In this the age of specialization it has acquired a special meaning. Without doubt clinical medicine – on which the greater part of modern medical research is built – is only one small area in comparison to the human task which falls to the healing arts as a whole. In this sense our title reveals a double aspect. On the one hand we have philosophy, the mother of all the sciences.[2] The expression 'the philosophical dimension' makes me aware of that peculiar isolation into which the need for solitude brings the reflective thinker. In Heidelberg there is a path called the Philosophers' Way which some people genuinely imagine was so named in honour of the discipline of philosophy. In fact this path bears its name by virtue of those remarkable people who prefer to go out walking on their own. This is the genuine origin of the name and indeed anything else would be too much honour for us philosophers. In the modern era, in the wake of Rousseau, it is the desire to go walking alone, to think alone, which invites us all to take up philosophical reflection. Nature is the animating spirit of such solitude. And then on the other side we have 'practical medicine', the waiting room, the white coat, the concern for every patient awaiting attention. It is not easy to throw a bridge from one bank to the other, for all the countless bridges which already span the Neckar. It is clear that philosophy must recognize just how remote it is from the sphere of praxis.

How then do things stand with this double aspect governing the relation between theory and praxis? In this question we immediately recognize one of the oldest problems affecting the ethical life of human beings. 'Theory' literally means observation, simply looking on, perceiving how things are or reveal themselves to be. It means not being persuaded by our own desires and interests to construe reality in terms of how we would like the world to be. In contrast to theory stands the world of praxis where every mistake revenges itself and where a permanent process of learning and self-correction is sustained through the experience of success or the lack of it. How are these two related to one another? How is it that we are able to adopt a strictly observational attitude towards things such as illness and death which are of such urgent importance to us? How is a productive relationship between theory and praxis to arise? I think it is important for us to be clear how difficult this has become for us all, especially since modern science has been forced to relinquish that unity which once existed between medical practice and our everyday lives. In earlier times there was the medicine man or the wise woman in the village. And then there was the almost paternal role of the family doctor. In smaller social structures there was a form of local praxis which did not expose the anxious patient to white coats and wearisome waiting rooms. But we live in the age of institutions and mass society. Science itself has become one such all-encompassing institution. Yet we must not deceive ourselves. There is no going back. What we need to do is to learn to build a bridge over the existing divide between the theoretician who knows the general rule and the person involved in practice who wishes to deal with the unique situation of this patient who is in need of care.

I need only call to mind what language itself tells us when it links science and art so intimately that the science and the art of medicine become peculiarly interfused. The term 'art' seems to belong to that domain in which someone's skills and abilities enable them to construct something, to 'make' something. And yet we all know that the task confronting the doctor is to 'treat' the patient, and hopefully to help bring about recovery. This is not the typical way of modern science, which has learnt to erect constructive models on the basis of experience, experiment and correct quantitative calculation. With medical practice we clearly find ourselves in a domain which requires us to apply what we have learnt in a very different manner. Once science has provided doctors with the general laws, causal mechanisms and principles, they must still discover what is the right thing to do in each particular case, and this is something which hardly seems to be predictable or knowable in advance. Clearly we are here concerned with a task of a quite different nature. But how is this task to be met?

Once again I shall begin my reflections by focusing on language. I am interested in the way in which we speak of the general relationship between a rule and a case. We say that something is a *case* of a regularity or a principle. But is the 'case' of a patient the same thing? For the patient who is suffering this 'case' reveals a quite different dimension. The 'case' of a patient is primarily a matter of disfunctioning, a condition of being excluded from the social world in which one actively lives and works. For the doctor too the 'case' of a patient is something quite different from what counts for science as the case of a rule or a law. Both of these meanings reside, as it were, within the same word: on the one hand, the particular instance of a rule, and on the other, the 'case' of an illness, which represents a completely different problematic in our experience of life and defines the exceptional position of the patient.

I am concerned with the question of why it was necessary for us to advance beyond that prescientific stage of knowledge and experience which, in many cultures and long before modern science, none the less provided a form of conduct and care for the sick and the dying. What is specific to our present situation, how has it become what it is, and what possibilities does it hold out to us? How is modern science to resolve this general problem and how should it address the specific problems which doctors face in contemporary society?

But medical science is not only concerned with illnesses, for illness cannot exist without health. Both of them belong to what a doctor must know or seek to know through the means of modern science. Here we are confronted with the still unanswered question: what is health? We know, roughly, what illness is. It is that 'revolt' or rebellion which takes place when something starts to disfunction. It thus appears as something set over against us, as an 'object' (*Gegenstand*), as that which offers resistance (*Widerstand*) and must be broken. We can examine an illness closely and evaluate its particular degree of virulence. And indeed we can do so with all the different means provided by the objectifying scientific method which we have acquired through the modern natural sciences. But health is something which somehow escapes all this in a unique way. Health is not something that is revealed through investigation but rather something that manifests itself precisely by virtue of escaping our attention. We are not permanently aware of health, we do not anxiously carry it with us as we do an illness. It is not something which invites or demands permanent attention. Rather it belongs to that miraculous capacity we have to forget ourselves. But then what does theory, this pure 'looking on', seek to discover? What does it find? Here we speak of the problem of the body and soul. We are confident that we know what the body is, but nobody knows what the soul is. What is the relationship between the body and the soul? Some kind of dynamic interrelationship perhaps? We can say that the body is life, that which is alive, and that the soul is what enlivens or animates. Yet both are so profoundly interrelated that every attempt to objectify either of them without the other in the end leads to absurdity. This serves only to reveal how great the distance is between what objectifying science is able to achieve and the task we are attempting to address here.

I am reminded of a passage from Hegel: 'The wounds of the spirit heal without leaving scars.' But this interesting idea needs to be expanded, for is it not a miracle of nature that it too knows how to heal without leaving scars behind? Convalescence, becoming well again, is a process of returning once more to one's accustomed form of life. In this sense the doctor is only somebody who helps along what nature itself must bring about. One of the sayings of the Greek physician Alkmaion runs: 'We human beings must die because we have not learnt to connect the end with the beginning again and this is something we can never accomplish.' This is a genuinely disturbing observation for it tells us that it is not something in particular that we lack, but rather everything. Only the vital, animating force of nature is able to do this, to return from the end of illness back to the beginning, through all the afflictions and diseases with which the body is assailed. Here as Alkmaion observes 'Death itself is simply a return into the cycle of nature.' When Alkmaion defines the mortal passing away of the individual as the inability to complete this cycle of return, he is clearly thinking in terms of the miraculous example of nature's own capacity for self-renewal. What wisdom is contained in this thought of an assimilation which is not properly described as dying!

Now, keeping this in mind, let us ask what it is that modern science does. Thanks to Galileo and the radical new departure initiated in the seventeenth century, science is now conducted in a completely new way. Modern science is characterized by its capacity, based on the mathematical model, to organize concrete information concerning observed phenomena under general laws. In this way it has developed a marvellous and astonishing ability to articulate and control important factors within specific fields of human experience to such an extent that it can even produce healing effects through the introduction of entirely new factors. The development of constructive models which allow the fundamental features of a universal principle to be grasped in its concrete instances undoubtedly represents one of the decisive achievements of modern science. But it is also clear that not everything can be achieved by such means. We also need something from the self-healing power of nature and of spirit. By the term 'spirit' here we need not think of anything too elevated. Let us say that spirit is both the body and that which animates it. Both together represent the spirit of our particular form of life, that which we all are, including both the patient and the doctor who helps the patient. Here it is clearly a question of learning to translate the skills through which scientific knowledge is object-ively applied into the other dimension where this animating force is sustained and renewed.

Everyone will immediately accept this as obvious. Clearly this is the task. The question is, how is it to be realized? For modern science to objectify something means to 'measure' it. Through experiment and by means of quantitative methods various vital phenomena and life functions are, in fact, measured. Everything is measured. We are even so bold as to establish so-called standard values, clearly one of the principal sources of error in established medicine. Instead of learning to look for illness in the eyes of the patient or to listen for it in the patient's voice, we try to read it off the data provided by technologically sophisticated measuring instruments. Both are perhaps necessary, but it is difficult to practise both together.

Once we start to think in this way we are obliged to ask ourselves what 'measure' actually means here. I value Plato's thoughts on this matter very highly and I can only recommend the study of his work to those who wish to understand what it is they feel to be missing in the world of modern science. In one of the dialogues concerned with the role of the politician, Plato raises the highly topical question as to what distinguishes a genuine statesman from a mere functionary of society. Plato distinguishes between two different kinds of measure. The first is that which is used when one wants to take a measurement and the procedure is brought to the object from without. The second is the measure which is to be found within the object itself. The Greek expressions here are *metron* for the first sort of measure and *metrion* for the second. In German we speak of 'das Angemessene', of what is appropriate or fitting. What does 'appropriate' mean here? Clearly in the present context it refers to that *inner* measure which is pro-per to a self-sustaining living whole. And we do in fact experience health in this way as a condition of harmony or an appropriate state of internal measure. This was how the Greeks viewed it. Illness on the other hand we experience as a disturbance of the harmonious interplay between the feeling of well-being and our capacity to be actively engaged in the world. Looking at things in this way we can see that what is genuinely 'appropriate' is accessible through mere 'measuring' only in a highly restricted way. Rather, as I have already suggested, what is important above all is observing and listening to the patient. But we all know how difficult this is in our vast modern hospitals.

I shall attempt to go a step further. It is clear that we encounter two different forms of measure, one belonging to the domain of science, the other belonging to the totality of our being-in-the-world. We have developed a modern terminological language to describe those systems which effectively sustain not only our own biological organism but also the innumerable institutions and establishments which constitute our social world. What follows from this observation? Simplifying matters somewhat I would say that, on the one hand, through observation and the collation of data by procedures of measurement we are able to develop an almost mathematical knowledge of how illness can be influenced. On the other hand, there remains what we call *treatment*. The German term *Behandlung* is a rich and significant word for 'treating' people and 'handling' them with care. Within it one hears literally the word 'hand', the skilled and practised hand that can recognize problems simply through feeling and touching the affected parts of the patient's body. 'Treatment' in this sense is something which goes far beyond mere progress in modern techniques. Here it is not only a question of the skilled hand but of the sensitive ear which is attentive to the significance of what the patient says, and of the doctor's observant and unobtrusive eye which knows how to protect the patient from unnecessary distress. There is so much of importance which depends on just how the patient undergoes this treatment.

The reflections which I am putting forward here are the impressions of someone who stands at a certain distance from these things. Fortunately, I have only rarely been ill and have always received the best of care. But I am thinking above all about the very old and the chronically ill. The illness of such people is of special importance for medicine today since it provides a painful demonstration of the limits of technical medical skills. It is precisely in the treatment of the chronically ill and ultimately in the care we give to the dying that we are reminded that the patient is a person and not a 'case'. We know the routine formulas with which doctors normally fulfil their obligations towards their patients. But when doctors genuinely succeed in leading a patient back into his or her own life-world, they recognize that they are called on to provide help not just for one particular moment but over the long term as well. Here doctors are called on not merely to 'act upon' their patients but to 'react to' them by treating them in a proper manner.

Finally, I shall try to draw a conclusion which affects all of us. In my view chronic illness represents a special case of something which confronts us all as human beings. For we must all learn to treat ourselves properly. It is the tragic fate of our modern civilization that the development and specialization of scientific and technical abilities has crippled our powers to treat ourselves in this way. This is something we must recognize as characteristic of our modern and so altered world. I know very well how much one should value the role modern medicine must play. Here it is often a question not only of making someone well again but of sustaining their capacity to work. These are necessities of modern industrialized existence which we must all accept. What goes beyond this, however, is the 'treatment' which we carry out with respect to ourselves, our capacity to listen to and be sensitive to what takes place within us. In those moments when we are not disturbed by pain we are able to experience self-fulfilment among the myriad riches which the world offers to us. In these moments we are closest to ourselves. This too represents a form of 'treatment' and I am increasingly convinced that in our industrialized society we must do everything we can to increase the value placed on such preventative measures, in comparison with the importance normally placed solely on the dimension of cure. This is something which in the long run will prove decisive if we are going to cope with the changed living conditions of our technologized world and if we are to learn to revive once again those forces which can help us to discover and preserve what is 'appropriate', appropriate for oneself and appropriate for each one of us, namely that internal condition of equilibrium.

Both science and the technical application of scientific knowledge have led to a domination of the natural world to an unparalleled extent. We have now reached a 'limit situation' in which this knowledge, ultimately, has turned destructively against nature itself. But alongside such knowledge and such technical capacities which treat the world as an object to be dominated and as a mere field of resistance, there is another perspective from which the world can be considered. The former view sees in every object a form of resistance, something to be broken down and mastered through acquiring knowledge about it. But an alternative view is offered by the idea of the 'life-world', introduced into the philosophy of this century by Husserl. When in my youth I first came to philosophy the established 'fact' of science represented the last word and formed the basis of so-called theory of knowledge. But things change and today we are far more aware that all methodological science encounters limits with respect to what it can hope to achieve. It will, of course, always seek to overcome these limits and they cannot be prematurely fixed in any obscurantist way. But it seems to me that there are other kinds of limits which do need to be respected. Thus it can be argued that anyone who thinks of themselves simply as a 'case' cannot receive proper treatment and that doctors cannot help anyone over a serious difficulty or even a minor affliction when they do no more than simply exercise the routinized skills of their particular discipline. From both perspectives we are partners in a life-world which supports us all. And the task which falls to us all as human beings is to find our own way in the life-world and to learn to accept our real limits. For doctors this path involves the double obligation of combining highly specialized skills and abilities with participation in the shared life-world.

Notes

1 We are unfamiliar with Agathon's works for the theatre because they did not primarily involve dialogue, as is the case with most of the Greek dramatists who are known to us. His work represented a more musical form of dramatic art which could not be passed down in the same way.

2 Philosophy has, of course, long since lost this role but it will continue to exist as a human phenomenon for as long as there are thinking beings on this earth. Although philosophy has often been pronounced dead, it never seems to have suffered as a result.

8

On the Enigmatic Character of Health

It is important to reflect on matters which not only concern doctors in their sphere of professional interest or as part of their training but which concern us all. Which of us cannot recall that first alarming experience in early childhood when we were suddenly pronounced ill on the authority of our parents and made to stay in bed the next day? The accumulation of such experiences in later life suggests ever more clearly that it is not so much illness that is something special but rather the miracle of health itself.

I would like to take this as an opportunity to try to locate the theoretical and practical position of medical science within the larger context of this society of ours which has been so shaped by the development of modern science, and to ask further how we should orientate ourselves within our own lives towards the phenomena of sickness and health. It is undoubtedly the case that in the experience of sickness and health alike a more general problem reveals itself, one which cannot be confined to the particular position occupied by medical science among the modern natural sciences. I would consider it a great advantage if we were all to be more aware of the important distinction between scientific medicine and the art of healing. This distinction is ultimately that between a knowledge of things in general and the concrete application of this knowledge to particular cases. As such this is an elemental theme of philosophy and human thought and also something which has particularly occupied me in my own philosophical work under the title of hermeneutics. Clearly it is only the first, knowledge in general, which can actually be learnt, while the other must gradually ripen through experience and the development of one's own powers of judgement.

These reflections serve to place our concerns in a much broader context. Ever since the development of modern science, with its tense relationship with the concrete wealth of lived human experience, humankind has found itself confronted by special tasks and responsibilities. We live, on the one hand, in an environment which has been increasingly transformed by science and which we scarcely dare to term 'nature' any more, and, on the other, in a society which has itself been wholly shaped by the scientific culture of modernity. Here we must learn to find our own way. Yet we are surrounded by innumerable rules and regulations which ultimately all point towards an ever increasing bureaucratization of life. How, in the face of all this, are we to sustain the courage to determine for ourselves the course of our own lives?

It strikes me as extremely significant that in today's highly developed technical civilization it has proved necessary to invent an expression like the 'quality of life', which serves only to describe what has been lost in the meantime. In fact this expression reflects a fundamental and immemorial human recognition that each of us has to 'lead' our own lives, that we must decide for ourselves how we are going to live. This is not only true for Europeans, for those whose outlook has been shaped by the scientific world-view. It is a fundamental theme that arises even where religious rites and healing knowledge still determine the care of the ill under the aegis of leading figures and social groups such as wise women or medicine men. Here we are unavoidably confronted with the question of whether the accumulation of such experience has produced practices which have proved themselves in the past and still retain their validity, even if we no longer find them reliable or understand the reasons for their effectiveness. This situation was characteristic of the entire early period of the development of humankind and certainly extends beyond the specific domain of sickness and health. By addressing the broader questions surrounding sickness and health I hope to bring to light the fundamental tension which is particularly characteristic of our own scientifically grounded modern civilization. And this is something I have sought to suggest with the title 'On the Enigmatic Character of Health'.

If we are looking for a definition of medical science, then the one that presents itself most readily to us is 'the science of illness'. It is illness which imposes itself on us as something threatening and disruptive which we seek to be rid of. Thus the fact that in the German language the term *Gegenstand* – meaning 'object', literally 'that which stands over against us' – has eventually established itself seems to be wholly in accord with that sense of radical new departure which has dominated modern science since the beginnings of modernity in the seventeenth century. *Gegenstand* is a highly significant word. It means that which offers resistance (*Widerstand*), that which withstands our natural impulses and which we cannot simply incorporate into the order of our lives. What we esteem in science is that capacity for objectification which is fundamental to the acquisition of knowledge. First and foremost here is the ability to weigh and to measure. We can never wholly escape from the fact that scientific and medical experience is primarily orientated towards forcibly 'overcoming' the manifestations of illness. When confronted by illness we attempt, so to speak, to overcome nature itself. What we seek to do is to master the illness, to gain control of it.

Through modern science and its experimental methods we compel nature to offer up answers. But in doing so we inflict a form of torture on it. Such practices derive from the great breakthrough of the seventeenth century with the struggle to break free from outdated prejudices and to open up new domains of experience in all directions. Now we should be aware that it is no accident that the German word *Ganzheit* meaning 'totality' or 'entirety', so frequently used today, is a very modern verbal construct. This word was still absent from the lexicons of the nineteenth century. Only after the methodological thinking of the mathematical-experimental sciences had already established itself so strongly in the domain of the healing arts did it become possible to lose oneself in the labyrinthine paths of specialization without any orientation towards the whole. We are all motivated by the desire to establish the same methodological certainty for our knowledge which we associate with objectivity and the scientific attitude. Nor should we imagine that we can simply turn our backs on this development. Meeting here together I hope that we all share a common sense of the task which confronts everyone who takes science seriously, especially when we consider it in terms of this watchword 'totality'. This is something which it is important not only for every doctor and every patient to think about, but for all those who do not wish to end up becoming patients themselves – and this ultimately includes us all. Unfortunately, we are obliged to concede that the progress of science has been accompanied by a decline in our more general care for health and in preventative medicine in general.

This much, in any case, is clear. The German concept of 'wholeness' is an artificial expression which only became necessary and meaningful through the existence of its conceptual counterpart, 'specialization'. Specialization is the irreversible tendency of modern science in all its different manifestations. As we all know, the law of specialization is not confined to the development of modern medical science and medical practice. Scientific research in every discipline finds itself facing the same situation. Each of the different areas of scientific enquiry are methodologically separated off from one another, which makes it imperative that we struggle to forge new, interdisciplinary links between them. Those areas which are not fully amenable to techniques of methodological verification we term 'grey zones', a label not restricted to things that are simply irrational. A good example is astrology. Can anyone really explain how it is that on the basis of horoscopes such astonishing predictions can be made about human life which then prove true? Here we can be sceptical but at the same time we all have the right to judge from our own experience. In any case there are things which cannot be explained here. In fact there are innumerable examples of such areas where science cannot say precisely what a particular procedure actually brings about in practice. For a long time homeopathy has been recognized as one of these areas. Indeed, it was the more well-meaning among sceptical clinicians who termed it 'oudenopathy'.[1] They believed that medicines containing such low homeopathic doses had absolutely no effect and that they only proved themselves in practice and enjoyed the appearance of beneficial healing effects because they prevented the potential misuse of other, biochemical medications.

The fundamental fact remains that it is illness and not health which 'objectifies' itself, which confronts us as something opposed to us and which forces itself on us. In fact, we always describe something as a 'case' of illness. The German word for case is *Fall*. What does *Fall* mean here? The use of the word undoubtedly comes from the game of dice. From there it has entered into the language of grammar and the rules of declension. It refers to the role which 'falls' to a noun within a sentence. (The Greek for *Fall* is *ptosis*, which in Latin becomes *casus*). Similarly, illness is something which 'befalls' or 'falls' to us, something we experience as a chance or accident (*Zufall*). This is also what the Greek word 'symptom' means. In the Greek it is used to refer to the conspicuous features which generally appear with the onset of an illness. Once again we must address the fact that the real mystery lies in the hidden character of health. Health does not actually present itself to us. Of course one can also attempt to establish standard values for health. But the attempt to impose these standard values on a healthy individual would only result in making that person ill. It lies in the nature of health that it sustains its own proper balance and proportion. The appeal to standard values which are derived by averaging out different empirical data and then simply applied to particular cases is inappropriate to determining health and cannot be forced upon it.

I use the term 'inappropriate' (*ungemäß*) intentionally in order to make clear that the application of rules on the basis of prior measurements is not something we naturally do. Measurements and the criteria and procedures by which we arrive at them depend on conventions. It is in the light of these that we approach the object of enquiry and subject it to measurement. But there is also a natural form of 'measure' which things bear within themselves. If health really cannot be measured, it is because it is a condition of inner accord, of harmony with oneself that cannot be overriden by other, external forms of control. It is for this reason that it still remains meaningful to ask the patient whether he or she *feels* ill. One has the impression that factors deriving from some of the most elusive experiences of life somehow come into play with the skills of a very gifted doctor. It is not only the scientific progress of clinical medicine or the ever increasing introduction of chemical methods into new fields of biology that serve to make a great doctor. These are all important forms of advanced research which make it possible to extend the domain where medical assistance can be given into areas where medicine previously was quite helpless. But the healing arts involve not only the successful struggle against illness but also the process of reconvalescence and, ultimately, care for health in the broadest sense.

I would like once again to turn to our use of language in order to illustrate what is meant by this inner proportion, this inner correspondence that cannot be measured and yet must always be taken into account. The role of the doctor is to 'treat' or 'handle' the patient with care in a certain manner. The German word for treating a patient is *behandeln*, equivalent to the Latin *palpare*. It means, with the hand (*palpus*), carefully and responsively feeling the patient's body so as to detect strains and tensions which can perhaps help to confirm or correct the patient's own subjective localization, that is, the patient's experience of pain. The function of pain in the living body is to register through subjective sensation a disturbance in that harmonious balance of bodily processes which constitutes health. We all know how difficult it is – above all at the dentist – to locate exactly where the pain is coming from. This is why pain must be 'drawn out', as it were, sometimes even simply through the pressure of the doctor's hand. Those doctors who are able to do this are in possession of a true 'art'.

There is a famous story told about the great Doctor Krehl whose name enjoys almost mythical fame among all students of medicine in Heidelberg. The story itself possesses an almost myth-like truth. In 1920 when the electric stethoscope was introduced Krehl was asked by his students whether this represented an improvement. To which he replied: 'Well, the old stethoscopes were better for hearing with. But I cannot judge whether you have sufficient experience to benefit from them.' This is also the case with *palpatio*, with examination by means of the hand. Some-one who can do this properly is able to perceive something in the process and every good doctor must attempt to learn this skill.

I concede that it may sound rather academic and pedantic to claim that one should think of the 'hand' when one hears the word *Behandlung*. But the wisdom of scholars is not always nonsense and sometimes it is also worth being aware of such things. Now that the origin of the word *palpatio* is clear, let us ask what *behandeln*, treating people, actually means. Once again the living use of the term extends far beyond the specific domain of medicine. Without being doctors we none the less 'treat' one another well or badly. What do we mean when we say this? Clearly what is demanded is that we treat someone in the 'right way'. Does this mean that we fulfil a norm or follow a rule? In my opinion it means, rather, that we address the other person in the right way, that we do not force ourselves on them or compel them to accept something against their will, be it an external measure or a regulation. What is important is to recognize the other in their otherness, as opposed, for example, to the tendency towards standardization promoted by modern technology, the autocratic control of education by school authorities or the blind insistence on authority by a teacher or a father. Only by means of such recognition can we hope to provide genuine guidance which helps the other to find their own, independent way. Treat-ment always also involves a certain granting of freedom. It does not just consist in laying down regulations or writing out· pre-scriptions. For the doctor it is fairly clear what it means to say that someone is undergoing treatment with them. It involves a certain responsibility but at the same time a certain care which must recognize the freedom of the patient. No doctor can pre-sume to want to exercise control over the patient. Doctors should provide advice and help where possible and must always know that the patient only remains under treatment until the point at which a recovery is made.

Every treatment stands in the service of nature. Thus the expression 'therapy', which derives from the Greek, actually means 'service'. This too requires a skill or ability which must not only prove effective against the illness but must also be accepted by the person who is ill. Caution and consideration are an integral part of any treatment. Doctors must also be able to build up their patients' trust in their skills. In order to possess authority doctors must not simply try and play upon that authority. It is for this reason that we find it so disturbing when surgeons simply say 'We'll soon get rid of that.' This way of speaking is clearly understandable in light of the fact that modern surgery has actually become a very highly developed technical skill. And yet doctors know that they are dealing with a human organism here and surgeons especially must consider that it is sometimes a question of life and death that is at stake. What is perhaps of most fundamental importance is that the real task which doctors must fulfil is not actually to 'make' or in a sense to 'do' anything. The doctor can only make a contribution towards guiding health in a certain manner, towards helping the patient get better. But what then is health, this mysterious phenomenon which we all know and yet somehow do not know precisely by virtue of the miraculous character which attaches to being healthy?

Through discussing what is meant by the term 'treatment' I have attempted to clarify what it is that is demanded of doctors. Clearly treatment does not mean the attempt to master the life of another human being. However, to say that one has 'mastered' something has become a popular expression in the modern world, as for example when we learn to master a foreign language or, in modern medicine, when it is said that an illness has been mastered. Although it is quite correct to say this, the claim must nevertheless be qualified. Everywhere we are confronted by limits to what we can do. Thus we say quite correctly when we can do something properly: 'I've learnt to do that now.' But ultimately there is much more involved than this. Something is never just a 'case' of an illness. Perhaps it is not so very strange, although it is certainly disturbing, that when someone attends a large hospital today they lose their own name and are allocated a number instead. This has its own logic. It is necessary that the patient can be directed to a specific section of the hospital, for one goes to hospital precisely in order to be examined. Finally, it is revealed to the patient that he or she is a 'case' of something.

It is no accident that all of my preliminary remarks have dwelt on the experiences which one undergoes as a patient. Although our theme here today is 'the enigmatic character of health', we are still taking up our perspective on it from the standpoint of its opposite. Even when we say that we have succeeded in 'mastering' or controlling an illness, it is as if we are separating the illness off from the person involved. The illness is treated as if it possesses an independent existence which we must seek to destroy. This takes on a specific meaning when we think on a larger scale, as for example about the great epidemics which modern science has now virtually succeeded in mastering. We know that an epidemic is made up of all the many individual cases of those who have fallen victim to it and yet at the same time we are aware that it seems to possess a certain independent existence. We must attempt to counter the resistance offered to us by such epidemics, even if this only results in nature developing new forms to threaten us with. As a result of these reflections we must recognize that health always stands within a broader horizon of permanent jeopardy and potential disturbance.

No illness manifests itself in exactly the same way in every individual. Our particular weaknesses as thinking beings can play a contributory role here. One imagines that something is the matter. One somehow does not feel quite right. Anyone who has encountered difficulties at work knows at once that all sorts of somatic symptoms start to appear when things are not going smoothly in one's professional life. Here in Heidelberg the study of psychosomatic conditions has not been neglected. Such studies may prove generally beneficial in so far as doctors are becoming increasingly aware of the extent to which their work is dependent on the contribution made by the patient. Even the most tried and tested forms of medical intervention are now recognized to depend on individual factors which can be quite surprising.

It is not my task to speak about things which other people know better through their own experience. But in fact medicine is only one among the many different aspects of life in modern society which have been rendered problematic by scientific developments and the processes of rationalization, automatization and specialization. Specialization above all is necessitated by practical requirements. And yet when it begins to ossify into fixed and inflexible practices it can also become a problem. This tendency to let something ossify into a fixed habit is clearly rooted in human nature. And yet in the scientific culture of modernity this natural proclivity has developed into what is now a way of life. The life of each individual has now come increasingly to be regulated in an automatic manner.

So what genuine possibilities stand before us when we are considering the question of health? Without doubt it is part of our nature as living beings that our conscious self-awareness remains largely in the background so that our enjoyment of good health is constantly concealed from us. Yet despite its hidden character health none the less manifests itself in a general feeling of well-being. It shows itself above all where such a feeling of well-being means we are open to new things, ready to embark on new enterprises and, forgetful of ourselves, scarcely notice the demands and strains which are put on us. This is what health is. It does not consist in an increasing concern for every fluctuation in one's general physical condition or the eager consumption of prophylactic medicines.

It is the disruption of health that necessitates treatment by a doctor. An important part of the treatment is that the patient actually discusses his or her illness with the doctor. This element of discussion is vital to all the different areas of medical competence, not just to that of the psychiatrist. Dialogue and discussion serve to humanize the fundamentally unequal relationship that prevails between doctor and patient. Such unequal relationships represent one of the most difficult challenges which confront us as human beings. Think for example of the relationship between father and son or mother and daughter, or of the role of the teacher, the lawyer, the priest or of any professional person. Here we all know how important it is that within such a relationship both parties are able to come to mutual agreement and understanding.

We need only reflect that it is quite meaningful to ask someone 'Do you feel ill?', but that it would border on the absurd to ask someone 'Do you feel healthy?' Health is not a condition that one introspectively feels in oneself. Rather, it is a condition of being involved, of being in the world, of being together with one's fellow human beings, of active and rewarding engagement in one's everyday tasks. Let us try, none the less, to identify those contrasting experiences in which what is normally hidden actually shows itself. Even when we seek to measure health precisely, we are simultaneously aware that all such procedures must themselves be subject to critical examination, since the establishment of standard values can mislead us when it comes to the individual case. Where does this leave us? Once again, turning our attention to language can help point us in the right direction. We saw that in German there are strong etymological links between the terms for 'object', 'resistance' and 'objectification'. These words point precisely to those recalcitrant matters which intrude into our human experience of life. This is something we can visualize most vividly if we think of health as a state of equilibrium. Equilibrium is a condition of experienced weightlessness in which different forces balance each other out. The disturbance of equilibrium can only be redressed by the introduction of a counterforce. But with every attempt to redress the loss of balance through applying such a counterforce a new loss of equilibrium is threated in the other direction. Remember what it is like the first time one tries to ride a bicycle, with how much effort one leans against the lefthand side of the handlebars, only to lean hard against the right side when the thing threatens to tip over, finally ending up on the ground after all.

The attempt to maintain an equilibrium is a highly instructive model for the theme we are concerned with since it shows the dangers involved in all attempts at intervention. There is always the threat of doing too much. This is something which Rilke expresses beautifully in the 'Duino Elegies' where he speaks of how 'The permanently too little springs over into the empty too much.' This describes extremely well how equilibrium can be lost through being forced, through too powerful an intervention. Both the general care of health and the tested forms of medical treatment are characterized by an analogous experience. This should warn us against the unnecessary prescription of medicines. For it is incredibly difficult to discover exactly the right moment and the right dosage for such medical intervention. These reflections are bringing us closer and closer to what really constitutes health. It is the rhythm of life, a permanent process in which equilibrium reestablishes itself. This is something known to us all. Think of the processes of breathing, digesting and sleeping. The cycle of these three rhythmic phenomena helps to produce vitality, refreshment and the restoration of energy. We do not need to stay in and read as immoderately as Aristotle did; he said that 'One goes walking for the sake of the digestion,' but one can go for a walk for other reasons, or even without a special reason at all. (But that is the sort of person Aristotle was. It is said that he spent every evening reading. To prevent himself from falling asleep he read with a metal ball held in his hand and a metal basin below. If he did fall asleep, the metal ball would wake him up again and he would be able to carry on reading.)

However, we cannot actually hope to gain full control of these rhythmic functions which take place as an integral part of ourselves. We can observe their mysterious character particularly clearly in the case of sleep. This is one of the greatest enigmas we experience in our lives. Think of the deepness of sleep, of sudden awakening and the loss of all sense of time so that we do not know if we have slept for a couple of hours or the whole night. These are extraordinary things. The ability to fall asleep is one of the most inspired discoveries of nature or of God, this gradual drifting away so that one can never actually say 'Now I am sleeping.' Greater difficulties are presented by the process of waking up, or at least this is so with the unnatural lifestyle demanded by modern civilization. At the same time these rhythmic processes are what actually sustain us. Such things have little to do with the consumption of tablets and the conscious attempt to exert an influence on them.

All these reflections could be further developed to help us recognize in the hidden character of health the mystery of our nature as living beings. And what touches here on life also touches on death. Doctors especially, with their knowledge of human nature, are confronted with this double aspect of our existence. All doctors take the Hippocratic Oath. We all know what is at stake in this but we also know how the cultural apparatus of our civilization, the way death is experienced and the problem of prolonging life in the context of terminal illness inevitably lie on the doctor's conscience. Plato says at one point that it is impossible to heal the body without knowing something about the soul, indeed without knowing something about the nature of the 'whole'. The term 'whole' here is not intended as a methodological catchword. It refers, rather, to the unity of being itself. It is the 'whole' in the sense of the movement of the stars above and the changes of weather below, the rise and fall of the oceans and the living nature of the woods and fields. It is what surrounds and encompasses the nature of human beings that determines whether they find themselves in a condition of safe health or exposed to dangerous threat. Medicine seems to be a genuinely universal science, especially if this 'whole' of nature is extended to include the whole that is our social world.

A famous saying by Heraclitus can perhaps serve to bring our thoughts on this theme together. He said that 'The harmony which is hidden is always stronger than that which is revealed.' This is both immediately illuminating, and yet at the same time leaves a great deal unsaid. One thinks immediately of the delight given by harmony in music, of the pleasure produced by the resolution of a complex tonal development. Or perhaps, one thinks of the sudden flash of insight concerning a train of thought in one's mind. But Heraclitus' real meaning only really becomes clear when we think of the harmonious balance of the 'humours', as they were called in ancient medicine. The harmony of health displays its real strength where it does not leave us numbed and deadened, that disturbing effect revealed or produced by persisting pain or the debilitating rush of intoxication.

I come to the end. Philosophers face the task of leading us away from concrete things and yet, at the same time, bringing something genuinely illuminating to our attention. And here I hope to have clarified the connection between medical 'treatment' and the reference to the 'whole' or the 'totality'. It is not simply a question of the correspondence between cause and effect, or between intervention and success. Rather, I have been concerned with that hidden harmony which we must seek to recover and in which we discover both the miracle of reconvalescence and the mystery of health. Such harmony can be understood as a form of protected composure, of *Geborgenheit*.

I would like to end with the claim that human beings, like all other living creatures, must always defend themselves against constant and threatening attacks on their health. The entire mucous membrane system of the human organism is like a giant filter which intercepts everything which might damage or overwhelm us. None the less we are not in a state of permanent defensiveness. We ourselves are part of nature and it is this nature within us, together with the self-sustaining organic defence system of our bodies, which is capable of sustaining our 'inner' equilibrium. This is the unique interplay of functions which constitutes life. We can only oppose nature through being part of nature ourselves and through being sustained by nature. We should therefore never forget that both the patient and the doctor must join in acknowledging the role of nature if successful recovery is to be accomplished.

Note

1 'Ouden' comes from the Greek word for 'nothing'. Here it is used to indicate a placebo medication which 'does absolutely nothing'.

9

Authority and Critical Freedom

I have been asked here to speak about the concept of authority, but my contribution can only be that of a philosopher, that is to say, of someone who is called on to render an account of the concepts we use and who does so by drawing on what we all fundamentally already think. For this is something which is, so to speak, deposited in language, where it lies ready to be grasped. I shall begin, then, with a discussion of the word 'authority' and its semantic field.

I found the response of my secretary when I used the word 'authoritative' with the intention of distinguishing it from 'authoritarian' to be extraordinarily revealing. This word has been so completely driven out of use by the term 'authoritarian' that she had never heard it before. The current predominance of the word 'authoritarian' is highly indicative. We use the word 'authoritative' on those increasingly rare occasions when we accept a statement, a command or whatever without contradiction. In contrast, the word *autoritär* in the sense of 'authoritarian' is of very recent origin in the German language and was clearly adopted from the French. Its original use in German reflects an extraordinarily interesting and important phase of our political history. It was evidently introduced in this century at the end of the 1920s or the beginning of the 1930s by neo-conservative thinkers who were convinced of the weakness of the Weimar Constitution and of the need for stronger political authority, and struggled to bring such a change about. This was the so-called 'Tatkreis', to which, among others, men such as Hans Zehrer and Ernst Nikisch belonged, and which was pushed aside by the fateful events of the year 1933. It was Hitler's seizure of power which first gave the word 'authoritarian' its ominous tone. It became fused as it were with the concept of totalitarianism, itself undeniably a concept which represents an abandonment of the great European political heritage. Since Montesquieu, this heritage has involved an aspiration towards the idea of a constitutional state, that is, one characterized by the division of powers and the protection of minorities. In contrast, the concept 'authoritative' has a clear and, in its own way, timelessly valid meaning. For example, we can speak of someone making an authoritative appearance or of exercising an authoritative influence, as in the field of education, and here a positive accent is laid on the concept of authority. When we say that a teacher has no authority, we know that we are referring to something indispensable for the practice of teaching in the classroom. And inversely, we could not speak of anti-authoritative as opposed say to anti-authoritarian teaching. This would make no sense whatever, so indispensable is authority to the whole practice of education.

However, this line of thought is not one that particularly recommends itself to current opinion, and for good reasons. For we all stand on the ground of the modern Enlightenment, whose fundamental tenet was so powerfully formulated by Kant: 'Have the courage to use your own understanding.' This statement was directly aimed at the authority of the church and the prevailing political powers, and can essentially be seen as a valid expression of the virtues of a bourgeois class which had come of age and risen to political independence. In the realm of education the positive ring of the term 'authoritative' could still be sustained because children are clearly not yet autonomous responsible adults.

Now if we want to shed some light on the concept of authority, we must actually start out from the word 'authoritative' as this is rooted in the German linguistic consciousness. For what is surely decisive here is that we only call someone 'authoritative' if they do not need to invoke authority. The word 'authoritative' precisely does not refer to a power which is based on authority. It refers, rather, to a form of validity which is genuinely recognized, and not one which is merely asserted. This is expressed in the fact that, for obvious reasons, one cannot really say how authority is first acquired. Anyone who carries out certain measures, performs certain actions and makes certain proclamations precisely in order to obtain authority fundamentally desires power, and is already on the way to an authoritarian exercise of that power. Anyone who has to invoke authority in the first place, whether it be the father within the family or the teacher in the classroom, possesses none. This is something I can illustrate through the example of my own teacher, the famous representative of the Marburg School of neo-Kantians, the philosopher Paul Natorp. As a young teacher he never succeeded in gaining authority in the classroom. He had a weak voice and lacked a particularly impressive appearance. But for all that he actually became a famous philosopher, and as one of the leading members of the Marburg School he clearly was an authority, and this in the presence of such men as Nicolai Hartmann and Ernst Cassirer, Boris Pasternak, Wladyslaw Tatarkiewicz, Ortega y Gasset and T. S. Eliot.

Here we are concerned above all with the authority enjoyed by doctors. For this reason I would like to begin with an observation which I consider to be fundamental for everything that follows. And this is that we should not approach this problem in terms of the authority of the institution, that is to say, of the professional status of the doctor. Rather, what is important is the expectation of authority, one could even say the desire for authority, which the patient brings to the doctor. Authority is something which doctors have almost pressed upon them.

This can be illustrated by an amusing experience of mine. An opinion poll conducted during and after the cultural revolution which swept through in the wake of the new industrial revolution in the second half of our century, revealed that the standing of professors was still a rather high one. This was something I found as astonishing as it was gratifying until one day I learned from an experienced sociologist that what was actually at issue in this opinion poll and its results was not my own academic profession but that of the doctor. People's faith in the authority of doctors is expressed by the fact that in a hospital one asks for the 'professor'. What we should learn from this is that it is not so much the *potestas*, the position of power or the authority to issue commands, which lies at the basis of the call for authority, but rather a wholly different sort of expectation. It is an expectation concerning superior knowledge and the doctor's ability to help the suffering patient solely by means of this knowledge.

Here we encounter a moment of unalterable reality which is the product of nature itself. We must recognize that relations of superiority and inferiority do exist. The authority of the father rests on the fact that the child looks up to him like a god. This is something you know better than I. However, I once experienced something very indicative in this respect which reveals how this inferiority of the child, this desire to recognize authority, also expresses itself in relation to teachers. My five-year-old daughter was listening to a conversation at table in which the head of the Marburg Gymnasium said, concerning some matter or other, with surprise, 'I do not know anything about that at all.' At which my daughter leant over to me and whispered in my ear, 'Funny, that a teacher does not know.'

It is not only the stories of children or the testimony of the sick which reveal to us the need and the desire for authority. Allow me to tell another story. (Telling stories is something we philosophers resort to when we fear that our all too abstract and technical way of talking might bore our listeners.) As a classical philologist, which is what I became after finishing my doctorate in philosophy, I remember the following experience in the seminar of my teacher in classical philology, Paul Friedländer. I had interpreted a technical term which appeared in a work of Plato in a particular way and given my explanation for it. Friedländer answered, 'No it is not like that, it is like this and this.' To which I responded with a touch of bitterness, 'But how do you know that?' With a smile he replied, 'When you are as old as I am, you will know it as well.' He was completely right and in the meantime, since I myself turned fifty, I have come to know such things. I was once incautious enough, or rather perhaps courageous enough, to mention this story during a lecture in order to illustrate how authority, that is, the authority of an acquired inheritance of knowledge and competence, plays a particularly large and important role in the human sciences. A rather foolish member of the audience accused me, on this account, of authoritarian Stalinism. This example from my own experience reveals something deeply rooted in human nature: that even in a state of perfect enlightenment we cannot ground everything we hold to be true through strict proof or conclusive deduction. Rather, we must permanently rely on something, and ultimately on someone, in whom we have trust. Our entire communicative life rests on this.

We can find this connection mirrored in the etymological background to the concept 'authority'. The term is derived from Latin, from the history of the Roman republic, and describes the status and dignity ascribed to the Roman senate. It is an interesting fact of constitutional history that the *gremium* of the senators possessed enormous importance for the government of the Roman republic even though it possessed no power to issue commands, no *potestas* over the bearers of office. If we wanted to use a modern constitutional expression, we could say that at most it fulfilled the function of providing guidelines. The power to act lay with the consul, not with the senate. But it was the senate which enjoyed the authority.

If we begin by considering the origin of the concept in this way, what can we say that authority rests on? We must answer: simply in the importance of the counsel which the senate gave, that is, simply in the recognition of its superior insight.

It seems to me that this is the case wherever we encounter genuine authority. Genuine authority is recognized as involving superior knowledge, ability and insight. This holds in all those cases where authority possesses a positive meaning, the child in relation to the father, the pupil in relation to the teacher or the patient in relation to the doctor.

In our present scientific age it is undoubtedly true that authority is grounded in the superiority of that knowledge which has been accumulated and passed on by science as an institution. This is one of the major fruits of the modern Enlightenment. Liberation from faith in authority was indeed a fundamental driving force of the Enlightenment, since all individuals, so long as they were able to use their own understanding, were held to be capable of attaining knowledge. Descartes even began one of his most famous books with the paradoxical expression of his firm conviction that nothing in the world is so evenly distributed as the power of understanding. With this, of course, he wanted to say that in order to reach knowledge the most important thing was the method by which the understanding was employed. Now method and methodology are, in fact, the hallmark of science. But they possess a human background. The self-discipline which allows someone to keep to a method – against those inclinations, assumptions, prejudices and subjective interests which tempt all of us into believing to be true only what suits us – here claims its superior value and validity. It is on this that the true authority of science rests. None the less, even institutions of power that possess authority for this reason are not always accepted. This explains why the concept of critical freedom is often employed as the antithesis of authority. In truth, modern science represents an impressive embodiment of critical freedom that is to be marvelled at. But we should also be aware of the human demand that is placed on all those who personally participate in this authority: the demand for self-discipline and self-criticism, and this is an ethical demand.

If you will allow me just once to appeal to an authority, it will be in this case to the authority of Kant. The man who made the unconditioned validity of the moral law the foundation of his moral philosophy – in opposition to the utilitarianism and eudaemonism of the Enlightenment – also described the human form in which this unconditioned character of the moral law appears. This in its most vivid formulation is: you should never use others merely as means but should always recognize them as ends in themselves. This is a very strong demand, and one which conflicts with the insistent force of our own self-love. It requires respect for the other to enable us to meet this demand. But what is respect? Respect is a highly dialectical affect. It involves the recognition of the superiority, or at least the independent significance, of the other, but reluctantly! It is bound up with the humbling of oneself. Thus we use the phrase 'that commands my respect'. This is how we speak when someone has said or done something very positive in our eyes but which we had not expected from them. Now, if I respect another person this involves recognition of their freedom, but this itself demands that I am myself really free. I must be able to limit myself. All genuine freedom includes limitation, and this can even require a limitation of one's own authority. What is in question here is the character of genuine freedom. Freedom is often put forward as the opposite term to 'authority'. But just as authority can be misunderstood as mere power, as *potestas,* so too freedom can be misunderstood if it is taken in turn to be the simple opposite of authority. Here it becomes dogmatic freedom. Dogmatic freedom, we may say, is the desire for control which brings with it a false sense of certitude. Genuine freedom, on the other hand, is the capacity to criticize, and this capacity to criticize includes and is a precondition both of our own recognition of the superior authority of others and of others' recognition of our own authority. There is, in truth, no real opposition between authority and critical freedom but, rather, a deep inner interconnection. Critical freedom is the freedom to criticize, and the most difficult form of criticism is clearly self-criticism. The distinguishing character of human beings, the ability to recognize our own limits, is based on this. It is the foundation of all genuine authority. The most immediate expression of self-criticism is our ability to ask questions. Every posing of a question is an admission of ignorance and, in so far as it is directed towards someone else, a recognition that they may possess superior knowledge.

Such fundamental moral-anthropological facts as these characterize the role of the doctor and the position doctors occupy between the authority they represent and the critical freedom they must retain. Doctors must also confront the temptation of wanting to play the authority, not only on account of the superior scientific knowledge and medical experience which they do enjoy, but also through the pressure of the patient's need for their authority. Psychiatrists and psychoanalysts are well aware of the temptation of suggesting their own ideas to the patient instead of facilitating genuine self-liberation through the patient's own insights. This represents just one particular case in what is a universal human predicament. We are all tempted to misuse the authority we possess.

Finally, I would like to say one thing which is tangibly concrete. Anyone who is tempted to play on the institutional force of their authority rather than on genuine argument is always in danger of speaking in an authoritarian as opposed to an authoritative manner. It seems to me that the best way of preserving the proper use of one's authority lies in the critical freedom to make mistakes on occasion and to be able to recognize this fact. I would like to finish by expressing my conviction that such critical freedom towards oneself is one of the strongest factors in genuine authority and that we can actually use this freedom to control the potential misuse of authority.

10

Treatment and Dialogue

As my theme today I have chosen to discuss the two concepts
of treatment and dialogue which serve to characterize the realm
of experience that belongs to the art of medicine. In this I am
guided by the conviction that we should never wholly separate
our conceptual language from the experience which has been
sedimented in the words themselves and which can still make
itself heard in their everyday use. I consider the continuing relevance of the Greeks for the more developed stages of occidental
culture to lie in the fact that their words and concepts have
grown, as it were, directly out of the spoken language itself. It is
only in recent times, and above all through Heidegger, that we
have learnt to recognize the full significance of the transformation which Greek philosophical and conceptual language under-
went as it was interpreted in the Latin language. And we are only
now beginning to realize the significance of the fact that it was
Meister Eckhart and Martin Luther who first opened up a new
dimension in the German language for our thought and our
conceptual discourse.

Thus I too would like to begin by discussing the meaning of
words. Let us consider first of all the German word *Behandlung*,
which signifies the 'treatment' or careful 'handling' of a patient.
A doctor will recognize straight away something which is already

implied in this word. All treatment begins with the hand, with the *palpus*, by means of which the doctor physically examines the patient's body and feels the body tissue. It required a doctor to remind me of this connection! In the context of the patient the word has now taken on its more general meaning, as when people say that they are undergoing treatment with someone. In the same connection something very similar has also taken place with the expression 'practice', which derives from the Greek word *praxis*. For us medical practice signifies a sphere of professional activity and we no longer hear in this word the original meaning of an application of knowledge. Right up to today the white coat serves to symbolize the professional appearance of the doctor in his or her practice. Here I intend to take my orientation from a consideration of these two words, treatment and dialogue, and, above all, from the relationship in which they stand to one another. From the title of my paper, which brings these two terms together, you will have noted immediately that something decisive seems to be missing, namely any mention of diagnosis. This is after all considered to be the contribution of science: the establishment and interpretation of clinical data which will allow doctors to work out a course of treatment. But as the term 'consulting hours' already suggests, the dialogue between doctor and patient also belongs to the process of treatment. It is this dialogue which consitutes the area of common ground between doctor and patient from beginning to end and which is able to break down the distance which lies between them.

In choosing my theme I also intended to discuss the hidden character of health, and I think that these two areas fit well together. If we look first at what is involved in 'treating' someone, we can see that it is in no way simply a case of doing or producing something, even if we do speak of 'producing' the patient's health in the sense of restoring it. For an astute doctor or patient will always give thanks to nature when someone succeeds in recovering from an illness. Let us consider how we talk about treatment in other contexts. We say for example that we have treated someone, or that somebody else has treated us, well or badly. This always involves a recognition of the other individual's personal space and of their difference from ourselves. We say, for example, that we must treat someone with care, that we must be careful what we do or say to them. And this is true for everyone who is a patient. All patients must invariably be treated with care, both because of their neediness and because of their extreme vulnerability. In order to preserve this important recognition of distance, doctor and patient must gain some common ground where they can come to mutual understanding. Such common ground can only be provided by the dialogue they sustain between themselves.

In the modern world, however, the opportunities for doctor and patient to enter into genuine dialogue with one another are extremely limited. The local doctor who was virtually a member of the family is a thing of the past. And the so-called consulting hours are hardly favourable to developing a proper dialogue. For then the doctor is never really free. When the patient is waiting in the surgery the doctor is always responsibly preoccupied with discussing and treating the previous patient. Moreover, patients themselves are often preoccupied with their own anxious expectations, if not with the atmosphere of apprehension which pervades the waiting room itself. Any sort of closeness between doctor and patient has become an extremely fragile achievement. This is especially the case in today's modern hospitals. Patients are disconcerted at the outset by losing their own names and receiving numbers instead: thus in a modern hospital a patient can be called with the number 57 for example. This is perhaps a necessity required by our modern health service and I have no intention of criticizing it here. Nor am I in any position to do so. But this does all serve to reveal the difficulty of the task which faces both doctor and patient alike, if they are to succeed in developing a genuine dialogue which can allow the treatment to begin and be sustained throughout the whole process of recovery.

In discussing the theme of dialogue I feel myself to be relatively competent. My contribution to this theme in the realm of philosophy has been to stress the fact that language is only properly itself when it is dialogue, where question and answer, answer and question are exchanged with one another. The idea of speaking to someone else who is to respond is already implied in the word 'dialogue'. These two aspects are inseparable. Prince Alfred Auersperg would call this an 'intrinsic correspondence' and argues that it manifestly resides in the nature of language itself. Language is only fully what it can be when it takes place in dialogue. All of the different forms of language use can be seen as various modifications of the more basic form of dialogue, as slight shifts of emphasis in the interplay of question and answer. When we talk of feeling 'invited' to speak or of 'falling' into discussion, it is as if the dialogue itself were playing an active role in which both sides find themselves caught up and involved. In the realm of medicine, in any case, the dialogue between doctor and patient cannot simply be regarded as a preparation for or introduction to the treatment proper. The dialogue between doctor and patient must rather be seen as part of the treatment itself and as something which remains important throughout the entire process of making a recovery. This whole relationship is articulated in the technical expression 'therapy' which derives from the Greek *therapeia*, meaning 'service'. It does not at all imply that in treating people doctors simply exercise mastery of their craft. Rather, it suggests a relationship of respect and distance between doctor and patient. We await helpful 'service' from a doctor, who is there for more than simply to 'tell us something'. In this connection doctors expect something of themselves and also expect patients to make their own contribution as well.

In the modern world, which is a world largely dominated by science, the art of medicine has become something especially thought-provoking. Yet it was already so regarded by the Greeks. And already with the Greeks the art of medicine found it necessary to defend itself against the various other popular forms of healing knowledge already in force. We must not deceive ourselves about the fact that science, especially modern science with its many different areas of specialization, confronts certain limits from the outset. Yet the goal of the art of medicine is to heal the patient and it is clear that healing does not lie within the jurisdiction of the doctor but rather of nature. Doctors know that they are only in a position to provide ancillary help to nature. No matter how sophisticated our technical means of treating patients may become, we will always remain bound by the truth expressed in that old saying of medical wisdom: 'surgical intervention is only surgical intervention after all.' The validity of this saying extends far beyond the domain of surgery alone. It is important to be aware of the extent to which our civilization as a whole with its foundation in science and its myriad technical possibilities constantly tempts us to believe that we are able to do whatever we wish. We hear this in the surgeon's abrupt 'We'll soon get rid of that.'

Let us reflect on the most fundamental of questions and ask what contribution science makes to the art of medicine. The reason why I say that science only makes a 'contribution' is unproblematic and must be clear to everyone. We need only consider how paradoxically the whole process begins in the first place. The patient is asked what is wrong, or, as we say in German, what it is that he or she feels to be 'lacking'. The task, then, becomes that of locating what precisely is out of place. The entire vast apparatus of medical diagnosis today consists in the attempt to identify just this. Here I am only describing what our language itself tells us. These are matters of real experience which we all encounter as human beings, doctors as well as patients. In a certain sense the healing arts have always required some kind of apologetic defence, precisely because they do not represent any visible process of making or doing. In order to address this question I once took up an ancient tract of the sophists. This helped me to show the extent to which the ancient world was aware that physicians do not simply create a product when they succeed in healing someone. Rather, health depends on many different factors and the final goal is not so much regaining health itself as enabling patients once again to enjoy the role they had previously fulfilled in their everyday lives. It is only once this is achieved that one can talk of a full 'recovery', though of course this often extends beyond the doctor's sphere of competence and responsibility. From the condition termed 'institutionalization' we know how difficult reentry into everyday life can be, even for those who have effectively regained their physical health.

Clearly, diagnosis is a matter which belongs to science. However, the paradox remains that the doctor still has to ask the patient in what way he or she feels unwell. The condition of 'not feeling well' and the necessity for the doctor to question the patient directly testify to the fact that being ill involves a disturbance whose cause remains concealed. Here it is a question of not yet knowing precisely what it is that should become the object of investigation, something which at this stage the doctor cannot know. Now a modern doctor might well reply that modern medicine is in fact quite able to do this. One only needs to examine and to record all the various functional life-processes which take place in the body, and perhaps even in the psychological life, of the patient and then compare these results and sets of data with established standard values. But an experienced doctor knows that such a method can only provide guidelines and only supply a preliminary overview of medical findings. A certain caution is always required, along with a more considered examination which also takes into account the patient's condition as a whole.

Is it not remarkable that health conceals itself in such a peculiar way? Probably we should say that when we are in good health we are permanently supported by a deeper stratum of unconscious life, by a general sense of well-being. But this too seems to be something which is hidden from us. Is this state of 'well-being' really something in its own right, or is it merely a condition in which nothing hurts any more and in which pain and discomfort have been dispelled? Can we even conceive of a condition of permanent comfort and contentment? I must confess that I am rather disturbed by Aristotle's picture of a divine being permanently and uninterruptedly present to itself and able to enjoy both its own presence and that of everything else which is presented to its contemplation. Such a god cannot know, for example, what it is to awaken, that moment of first light when something actually becomes 'there' for us. It cannot know any of the things which are bound up with the dawning of a new day. Expectation, care, hope, the future – all these are involved in the process of waking up. And corresponding to this there is sleep and the process of falling asleep, which are marked by a particularly mysterious and obscure characer which borders on that of death itself. For no one can 'experience' their own falling asleep. What is contained in this constellation of sleep and death, of sinking into sleep and waking up again? I often think of some of Heraclitus' sayings concerning the proximity between sleep and death. In particular I recall the fragment which says: 'The harmony which remains hidden is mightier than the harmony which is revealed.' We can regard health as a miraculous example of such a strong but concealed harmony. When we are in good health we are genuinely absorbed in what we are doing, but we all know just how easily this heightened condition of wakefulness can be disturbed by the slightest discomfort and, above all, by physical pain.

From the work of Prince Auersperg, whose memory we are here to honour, I have learnt to understand the special form which pain assumes. He discusses the way in which pain is capable of claiming the whole of the self. But he also shows us that peculiar self-concealment which belongs to pain, so that it often proves difficult to say exactly where it hurts. It is by no means easy to tell the dentist which tooth is actually causing the pain or which one we suspect is the source of it. What must be concluded from all this within the context of the efficient application of medical knowledge is that more is demanded than simply recording data or, as we say today, 'checking' the different processes which take place in the body.

As an old Platonist I would like to recall a passage from the *Phaedrus* which expresses a genuinely Platonic thought:

SOCRATES: Rhetoric is to be considered the same as medicine.
PHAEDRUS: How so?
SOCRATES: In both cases there is a nature that we have to determine, the nature of the body in the one, and of the soul in the other, if we mean to be scientific and not content with mere empirical routine when we apply medicine and diet to induce health and strength, or words and rules of conduct to implant such convictions and virtues as we desire.
PHAEDRUS: You are probably right, Socrates.

SOCRATES: Then do you think it possible to understand the nature of the soul satisfactorily without taking it as a whole?
PHAEDRUS: If we are to believe Hippocrates the Asclepiad, we cannot understand even the body without such a procedure.[1]

Ancient medical writings are actually full of descriptions of the general surrounding conditions in which patients found themselves. Since then we have learnt even better to appreciate the extent to which good health requires a harmonious relationship consonant with both our social and our natural environment. It is this harmony which first enables us to move in accord with the natural rhythms which govern our bodily life. This is the case, for example, with the rhythm of breathing or with the cycle of sleeping and waking. Is the facility for collecting data which is so prized by modern science really adequate for grasping phenomena such as these?

Once again I would like to refer to one of the Platonic dialogues, this time *The Statesman*. Here Plato introduces two different concepts of measure and measurement. In fact, if we think back to the beginnings of modern science at the start of the modern period, we can see what an enormous transformation had taken place in our very concept of measurement even at this early stage. This can already be seen in the work of Nicholas of Cusa, who proposed whole programmes for measuring and quantifying phenomena, although it is true to say that by doing so he only hoped to discover more exact confirmation for old accepted truths.

In the meantime, however, modern science has come to regard the results of such measuring procedures as the real facts which it must seek to order and collect. But the data provided in this way only reflect conventionally established criteria brought to the phenomena from without. They are always our own criteria which we impose on the thing we wish to measure. This is something we have become accustomed to doing all the time and it is what doctors generally do when confronted with a new patient. And yet doctors treat themselves quite differently. When I asked a doctor friend of mine who had fallen ill what his temperature was according to the thermometer, he simply made a dismissive gesture with his hand. He never used the thermometer on himself and it was of no interest to him. However, there is another concept of measure which is distinct from the realm of the measurable. It is this we find in the Platonic dialogue *The Statesman*. Here Plato suggests that there is a form of measure which is not imposed on an object from without but which rather resides within the object itself. In the German language we can express this by saying that we recognize not only what can be measured externally (*das Maß*) but also what is 'fitting' or 'appropriate' (*das Angemessene*). What is appropriate cannot be ascertained through any act of measurement. Of course temperature can be measured, but only by comparing the recorded temperature with some standard norm, and this involves a crude process of standardization. The attempt to establish precise correspondence with standard values through medical intervention can actually bring about a deterioration in the patient's health. The true meaning of what is fitting or appropriate resides in its peculiar character as something which precisely cannot be defined. The whole system of self-regulating processes which take place in the body and in the human social environment possesses something of this 'appropriateness'. However, it is not in the science of medicine alone that the procedure of collecting data is accorded priority. For this is a product of the universal concept of method which is so closely bound up with the modern conception of science. One can almost say that it is the scientific method which first constitutes the object of knowledge. Everything which is not accessible to examination, which cannot be opened up to scientific method and so to regulation and control, is said to lie in the so-called grey areas where things cannot be treated with scientific exactitude.

The distinction which we have drawn between *metron* and *metrion*, between measure and what is measured on the one hand, and what is fitting or appropriate on the other, serves to reveal the degree of abstraction which is involved in the attempt to objectify phenomena through modern scientific methods of acquiring data. Max Planck once said that 'facts are what can be measured.' It is clear that both the concept of method and the concept of measure are related to the priority ascribed to self-consciousness in modern thought. At this point I would like to do a little more justice to Aristotle and remind ourselves that when he described the divine as a being which is permanently present to itself, he also added immediately that for us mortals such self-presence is only ever *en parergo*, something which occurs alongside other things. We are only able to become aware of ourselves when we are fully occupied with something else that is there for us; only when we are completely involved in something beyond us can we return to ourselves and become aware of ourselves. The ideal of complete self-presence and self-transparency that would correspond to the concept of *nous* or 'spirit' or the more recent concept of subjectivity is something fundamentally paradoxical. The state of being completely involved in something, of seeing it, intending it and thinking it, is necessarily presupposed if there is to be any possibility of 'returning' to oneself.

I have been particularly interested in this process of return in connection with the language of poetry. Poetic language always simultaneously involves a return to the actual sounds and marks of language. But such reflections do not belong here. To take up our present considerations once again, let us turn to the necessary limits of the objectification of experience. The German language helps to make this beautifully clear by offering two different expressions for the word 'body', *Körper* and *Leib*. When we use the term *Leib*, by virtue of a never fully eradicable feeling for language, we immediately associate it with 'life', with *Leben*. The living body and life are things that cannot simply be measured. But the term *Körper*, on the other hand, even in the broadest sense of the word, always refers to something which is readily susceptible to objectification and processes of measurement.

I do not consider it adequate to term everything which cannot be abstractly measured 'appropriate' (*angemessen*). For the statement that something is 'unmeasurable' only indicates a rejection of the reductionism implied in the scientistic interpretation of phenomena, and implies its own limitation. On the other hand, what is genuinely 'fitting' or 'appropriate' possesses a form of rightness which is wholly independent and which does not first need to be defined in terms of the negation of something else. Something similar is the case with the 'anti-logic' of perception, which was researched by Viktor von Weizsäcker. This is something I have learnt a great deal from. For here too it is necessary to free ourselves from abstract ideal constructions if we want to understand experience in an appropriate manner.

This is also the case with the concepts of the unconscious and the subconscious, though this is something of which I hardly dare to remind an audience of specialists. These are 'anti-logical' concepts, that is, concepts where one term can only be described in terms of the negation of the other. The reflections we have been pursuing here today are fundamentally concerned with the situation of the world as a whole. They are concerned with the task confronting our civilization of how to find a way back to what is 'appropriate', back to a situation in which the natural course of physical and organic life as well as of our mental and spiritual well-being can achieve a certain balance. Anything that can be objectified and made into an object has already been removed from that state of balance which characterizes the realm of nature. This is where something like 'appropriateness' belongs, that invisible harmony which, according to Heraclitus, is the mightiest of all and holds sway over all things.

It is in this broader context that I am interested in the experience of pain and, in particular, in Goethe's famous claim that he could not recall a single day in his life when he had not experienced pain. This was, of course, said by a man possessed of exceptionally acute powers of self-observation and heightened sensitivity. But the fact that he could say this testifies to the confident self-control with which he was able to overcome pain and bring himself back towards a feeling of well-being. There is a well-known and astonishing story about how Goethe at the age of eighty-one managed to survive a severe illness which had led his doctors to give up all hope for him. Suddenly, he demanded water. The doctors granted him this request only because his condition appeared fatal anyway, but the process of recovery actually began with this draught of water. No doubt today one could explain exactly the causal effects produced by the drink at this stage in the illness. I do not wish in the least to dispute the fact that modern research, together with its methods of acquiring scientific data and the rational application of such results, possesses a great deal of knowledge, far more than is known by lay persons such as myself.

But here I come to a point which has increasingly occupied me the older I have become. I think I also referred to it at the gathering in honour of Viktor von Weizsäcker. It is my opinion that the insights we have gained into the nature of psychosomatic conditions are of even greater importance to the patient than the doctor. We all need to learn once again that every disturbance in health, every complaint, however minor, and even every infection is actually a sign telling us that we need to restore what is appropriate, that we must regain the balance of equilibrium. Ultimately, both disturbance and the overcoming of disturbance belong together. This fact is constitutive of life itself. And it is this which places a critical internal limit on the concept of treatment. Every doctor who is treating a patient knows this only too well. Doctors must always hold themselves back in order to be able to guide their patients with a cautious hand and allow a patient's natural condition to restore itself.

Here we can see the significance of the dialogue between doctor and patient and the common ground it creates between them. This is quite the opposite of the mysterious Latin words which doctors sometimes whisper to one another when treating a patient and exchanging observations. Even if it is not always a case of using a word like *exitus*, I understand the reasons for this. A doctor will not wish to unsettle the defenceless patient, but at the same time does not want to have to forsake the opinion of other colleagues. However, a cautious hand is needed if the treatment is not to disturb and upset patients but, rather, is to succeed in helping them back on to their own two feet again.

The dialogue between doctor and patient is not only carried out in order to establish the patient's case history. That is a modified form of communication which belongs to the dialogue between doctor and patient principally because the patients want to remember and relate their own medical history. Sometimes it works out just as the doctor would like it to, and 'patients' are able to forget that that is what they are and that they are undergoing treatment. If patients succeed in taking up the same sort of dialogue as they would normally pursue when trying to reach agreement with someone, this can help to stimulate the ongoing process of easing the relationship between pain and well-being, as well as the experience of regaining equilibrium. In the somewhat tense relationship between doctor and patient, dialogue can help a great deal. But this dialogue is only really successful when it takes place almost as if it were a normal conversation. In our everyday lives we fall into discussions which are sustained by everyone involved rather than led by one person in particular. And this is how it should be even for the special form of dialogue that takes place between doctor and patient. In Plato's Socratic dialogues it appears as if the dialogue is always led by Socrates. The other partner in dialogue is often scarcely noticeable. But even here it is precisely through such dialogue that the other is to be brought to a point where he is able to see things for himself. Eventually he finds himself in an aporetic situation in which he no longer knows what to answer. But even where Socrates enumerates all the defining elements of a problem, this does not have the character of simple instruction, of an attempt to dominate the other as if Socrates knew everything. Genuine dialogue, rather, is concerned with creating the opportunity for the other to awaken his or her own inner activity – what doctors call the patient's own 'participation' – without losing their way once again.

It is precisely through the school of phenomenology founded by Husserl that we have learnt the importance of recognizing what each of us must see for ourselves. In my opinion it is a highly questionable development that technological forms of thought have begun to invade our use of language and that we now try to conceive of language as a form of rule following. I do not dispute that there is a great deal in the living use of language that can be described in this way and we should not underestimate the possibilities for expression which are opened up by that unconscious rule-following which belongs to linguistic competence. But the real miracle of language is to be found where someone – perhaps contrary to all prescriptions – succeeds in finding exactly the right word or discovers the perfect expression in the words of someone else. It is this which then proves to be the 'right' thing. In the background of our own discussions today I would like to see the emerging possibility of reintegrating the theoretical discipline which is required in science with those other motivating forces which we describe in terms of 'practical reason'. Since the eighteenth century this is the term we have used to describe what the Greeks meant by the words *praktike* and *phronesis*, namely an awareness appropriate to a particular situation, like that in which diagnosis, treatment, dialogue and the participation of the patient all come together. What takes place here between doctor and patient is a form of attentiveness, namely the ability to sense the demands of an individual person at a particular moment and to respond to those demands in an appropriate manner. It is in these terms that we must understand what is involved in therapeutic dialogue. It is not properly a dialogue in the sense in which we have been discussing it today, since its first aim is to attain its goal through dialogue. It is an attempt to set in motion once again the communicative flow of the patient's life experience and to reestablish that contact with others from which the person is so tragically excluded.

Thus the mystery of health remains concealed. This concealment belongs to the preservation of good health and this consists in forgetfulness. One of the most important healing powers in our lives resides in the ability every evening to sink into the healing sleep of forgetfulness. Not to be able to forget is a severe affliction. It is not a skill that lies within our power. Perhaps you will allow me to tell an amusing story here. It concerns an alchemist and supposedly took place in Dresden, where porcelain was invented around the time when attempts were still being made to transform base metals into gold.

There was once an alchemist at court who was very highly paid. After many, many months the sovereign who was employing him lost patience and finally demanded to see results of some sort. The alchemist replied that everything was ready for the experiment. The whole of the court gathered to witness it. But before the experiment began the alchemist announced: 'There is just one condition which everyone present must fulfil. During the experiment no one must think about an elephant.' Here we learn, if we did not know it already, what it means to be told not to think about something. The joke is a perceptive one. What stands behind it, of course, is the recognition that it is actually impossible to make gold. But to be able to forget, as if this were a skill one could master, is equally impossible. The limits of what can be mastered do not constitute the entire significance of what supports and sustains our lives. This is true for each individual, for society as a whole, for the relationship between all the different societies in the world, and for our relationship to nature. We all find ourselves constantly travelling on the same path. There are limits to what we can know and there are limits to what we can do. Knowledge – and not only the knowledge of science – is power and enables us to control things. Humankind must assert itself against nature as well. It is the unique situation of human beings that through our own conscious choice we are forced to assert ourselves. As human beings we are not wholly accommodated to our natural environment through the mechanisms of instinct and reaction. Precisely this is our 'nature', that we must assert ourselves over and against nature as far we can. But it is also and especially in the nature of human beings, in all they know and do, to sustain a relation of harmony with nature. This belongs to the most ancient wisdom of the stoics. Does it hold true only for the philosophers? I do not believe so. I always feel uncomfortable when people expect the philosopher to be presumptuous enough to claim to know what nobody else recognizes or understands, or even to know better than anyone else what first needs to be done. In my opinion philosophical thinking simply consists in making what we all already know another step more conscious. But this means, too, that philosophers do not know everything and this recognition itself leaves us that much less likely to be tempted to misuse the knowledge and skills we presume ourselves to possess.

Note

1 *Plato's Phaedrus*, trans. and with introd. and commentary by R. Hackforth (Cambridge and New York, 1952), 270bc.

11

Life and Soul

It remains important for everyone who pursues psychology to concern themselves with philosophy, and above all with its earliest beginnings in the thought of the Greeks. This is something I hope to show in the course of this lecture. The theme which I have chosen, 'Life and Soul', is admittedly an extremely difficult problem. One can only respond to it as did Socrates, with the words 'ou smikron ti', 'that is no small matter.' You will notice that I do not continue my discussion of this theme by directly addressing the topics of 'consciousness, self-consciousness and the mind', which on a certain preconception of the matter could count as an enumeration of all the things which connect the discipline of psychology with that of philosophy. But there clearly no longer exists anything like a discipline resembling philosophical psychology. This came to an end with Kant's famous critique of the *psychologia rationalis* and, in particular, with Moses Mendelssohn's magnificent reworking of Plato's *Phaedo*. Whether the immortality of the soul can be proven through concepts alone, as Mendelssohn attempted to do in his bold reinterpretation of the *Phaedo*, is no longer an issue of contention. Even German Idealism was concerned with a fundamentally different problem when it attempted to reintegrate psychology along with all the other sciences back into philosophy. The project which

Schelling and Hegel undertook was in a certain sense hubristic, and it produced a counterreaction on the part of the empirical sciences in the nineteenth century which finally threatened to reduce philosophy to a form of psychology.

I come from Marburg, where one of the great occasions in German academic life took place when the leader of the Marburg School of neo-Kantianism, Hermann Cohen, stepped down and together with Erich Jaensch was called to take up a chair in experimental psychology. At the time this struck everyone as a sensation, and in fact it did represent a significant moment. However, psychologists and philosophers would now agree that philosophy should not be dismantled in this way and that separate chairs in psychology should be created. But in so far as the themes of consciousness and self-consciousness remain absolutely central both to philosophy and to experimental psychology, the empirical inheritance of German Idealism can be seen to have left deep traces. In fact the entire intellectual history of the nineteenth century can be seen as a continual transgression of the limits of consciousness by those thinkers who made this a central theme, such as Schopenhauer, Nietzsche and Freud. It was not only in the phenomenon of dreams but with the help of dreams themselves that the entire nocturnal world which we call the world of the unconscious was opened up as a field of study. The very expression 'the unconscious' provides ultimate proof of the extent to which nineteenth-century thought was dominated by the notion of consciousness. Thus there is already a sort of admission contained in my choice of the title 'Life and Soul' for my theme today. Anyone who knows something about antiquity will be aware that for the Greeks these two words possessed almost exactly the same meaning. It is only in our century that the concept of 'life' has taken up a position at the centre of philosophical enquiries.

We do not in fact know what is really meant by the word 'soul', a word in which so much experience has been sedimented. No really persuasive etymology of the word soul has ever been put forward and it does not belong to that same family of words which in other languages has yielded *animus*, *anima*, *l'âme* and so forth. The fact that in today's modern psychology the terms 'life' and 'soul' are still used to refer to something specific is highly revealing. The phenomenological turn in philosophy contributed importantly to the attention which has been given to these phenomena. Figures such as Edmund Husserl, Max Scheler and Martin Heidegger, as well as those involved in the study of philosophical hermeneutics, have all made contributions in this direction.

Perhaps we should therefore pay more attention to the sedimentation of individual and worldly experience which resides in words themselves. I would like to place two German words, *Leben* (life) and *Leib* (the body) in the foreground. The meaning of both of these terms can be heard in the Greek word *psyche.* Everyone can hear the connection that exists between *Leben* and *Leib*, and indeed the two words are linguistically very closely related. In the Germanic language they were originally one and the same word. In the Greek word *psyche* we hear the same connection. It refers to the breath, to respiration, to that intangible something which separates in an inimitable manner the living from the dead. The Greek language possesses two different expressions for life, *zoe* and *bios*, both of which are borrowed into German to construct new words. It is not easy to differentiate them clearly from one another and yet we all know that we mean something quite different by 'zoology' than we do by 'biography'. This distinction already provides us with the most important insight, that is, that *bios* refers to a life that interprets itself, or one which can be 'understood' by others.

If, on the other hand, we start out from the assumption that we are concerned here with the body, with breath and the process of respiration, then our investigation into these words leads us towards consideration of a fundamental problem which is now a concern of modern neurophysiology, just as it has been of philosophy since time immemorial. I refer to the still highly relevant problem of the power of self-movement. One does not really need to be a philosopher to recognize that one of the most important attributes of all living things is the capacity for self-movement. Greek philosophy also described the living being as *heauto kinoun,* that which moves itself. Consideration of this phenomenon obliged

Aristotle to make the most subtle conceptual distinctions. For here we are forced to ask about the nature of something which is otherwise unknown in our experience: nothing moves unless there is something else which moves it. This seems so obvious that it is a consciously paradoxical formulation to speak of an 'automobile'. And in fact modern neurophysiology considers the perception of our own self-movement to be quite different from our perception of being moved through something else. It is a demand placed on thought itself to attempt an approach to the mystery of the living being in terms of this problem.

Taking our clue from the linguistic connection between breath, respiration and life, we can perhaps characterize what is specific to human nature in a different way. The Pythagoreans, at least, already connected the concept of *psyche* with that of *anamnesis*, with the realm of memory and of recollection. The Greeks made a number of different attempts to grasp this phenomenon. I call to mind how in Plato's *Phaedo* the periodic cycle of natural phenomena is considered inadequate to explain the fate of the soul and the question of immortality and how Socrates and his partners in the dialogue make reference to our ability to recollect what we have once seen, and so to the mysterious capacity for thought itself.

The capacity for thought introduces us into a new dimension of being. But what do we mean by this? We speak of *mneme* and *memoria*, both of which are firmly programmed among the characteristic traits and instincts of all living creatures. But *anamnesis*, the capacity for recollection, is clearly something different. It does, of course, have something to do with *mneme*, with memory, but it also seems to be something reserved in a specific way to humankind. Recollection, *anamnesis*, is a form of thinking, of *logos*, and that means it is connected with searching or inquiring. We all know what it is like to have a word on the tip of our tongue and yet to have to struggle to find it, often failing to find exactly the one we are looking for. But that we can seek after something in this way and finally recognize it when we have found it, this is a characteristic of what it is to be human. Hegel invented some powerful and vivid images to depict this dimension of being. He spoke of the 'night of preservation'. This is the realm of *mneme* into which everything which has been experienced sinks down and loses its presence – and yet, without ever being fully present, can none the less be repeated once again. In this way the 'night of preservation' is mysteriously related to the specifically human power of being able to bring back what has sunk down. Such an ability finds itself already on the way to language.

What then is this power and what is it able to achieve? The Greeks ventured the first steps in coming to an understanding of this. In one of Plato's dialogues, the *Charmides*, there is an interesting passage where I believe I can detect a reference to Heraclitus. The passage is concerned with how *dynamis*, 'power', is always a power to do something. But can someone have a power over themselves? What would it mean to have power over oneself? We are somehow aware that all the different powers we possess are, in fact, always already powers over ourselves. Perhaps this is actually the defining characteristic of things such as 'self-movement', that they too are a form of power which something can be said to possess over itself. Is this not something which we experience every morning, the awareness of self-movement, the upsurge of vital energy, the sudden illumination of presence? Between death-like sleep and suddenly being awake, two things which are so distinct from one another, there is a mysterious absence of transition. We do, of course, sometimes say that we are only 'half awake'. But we are fully awake even when we are half awake. This was the theme which concerned Heraclitus. How is it that waking and sleeping, and life and death, represent an indissoluble unity and are connected to one another without any intermediate stage between them?

If we were to describe what it means to have a power over ourselves, we would perhaps say, 'I am aware of my own powers.' Once again we are engaged with the concept of consciousness, which under the term 'reflection' dominated the thought of the last century. Reflection is a Latin word which was taken into the German language. It was originally used in the context of optics and our first knowledge of it comes from Stoic philosophy; it described the mystery of light as consisting in the fact that in lighting up everything else it thereby illuminates itself as well. And indeed light without reflection would be equivalent to night. For all observation is completely dependent on the reflection of light. The concept of reflection became firmly established in philosophical thinking in the modern period and here I come to the decisive complex of problems. What I have just been speaking about were the groping attempts of a highly gifted speculative culture to grasp mysterious marginal phenomena such as sleeping and waking and the hiatus between life and death with the vocabulary which the Greeks formed from out of their actual observation of the world. It is here that we must locate the mystery of consciousness and the problem of self-consciousness. Clearly what we are speaking about now is the soul, but what is the soul and what is the form of thinking which first comes to pass with the existence of humankind? For the Greeks clearly taught that there can be no thinking without the existence of the soul.

But what do we mean by thinking? The Greeks spoke of *nous*, by which they originally meant the immediate evidence of what we have before our eyes, whether this is seen with the real eye or with the inner eye which mathematicians possess when, instead of simply seeing the actual shape in front of them, they perceive the true triangle as it were in and through the shape. This is something which we all do, in fact, whenever we use words to communicate with each other. We retrieve words from our memory and through them we are able to see something before us just as mathematicians are able to see figures. Thus *nous* came to be regarded as 'pure' thought. For this reason Hegel was able to rediscover the highest form of thinking, self-consciousness, in Aristotle's *Metaphysics* where *nous* is used to characterize the divine being which moves the whole of nature. In order to describe the dimension of pure thought, Plato's Socrates takes over the idea of *anamnesis* from the soteriological doctrine of the Pythagoreans concerning the transmigration of souls. Socrates shows that the activity of recollection is something which we are all permanently involved in whenever we are engaged in thinking. It is only because we already have an intimation of something that we seek to bring it to mind and eventually discover what it was that we were actually looking for. In this way the dimension of the past is opened up to us and we develop a sense of time itself. We are able to conceive of a plurality of different possibilities among which we then have to choose. This is also the case with recollection. We try to remember something and often it is only by making an effort that we succeed in identifying it from among the flood of ideas and images which press in on us. This is what is involved in thinking, in moving back and forth in deliberation (*logizesthai*). And this is what is meant by the 'soul', for the soul is permanently 'concerned' with something. The expression for this in the *Phaedrus* is *epimeleia*. Concern, however, is never something internal and self-contained since we are always concerned about something or for somebody. Only in this way can there be concern for oneself and also what we have termed the power over oneself which is peculiarly characteristic of human *nous*.

Aristotle had great difficulty in finding the appropriate place for the concept of *nous* in his *Metaphysics*. And this means finding the appropriate place for it within the framework of a study of 'physics', within the order of beings. Aristotle sought to combine the concept of pure, godlike thought with the religious tradition of the Greeks, and for this reason described *nous* by virtue of its independence, its self-reflexivity and its self-referential character as the highest mode of being. To be nothing but complete self-absorption, to be dependent on nothing and to include everything in itself – this is what it is like to be divine. But how can this still be called thinking? Thinking is always the thinking of something and only a being who thinks something can become aware of itself. From the language and life-world of Greek thought Aristotle only had the terms 'doing' and 'suffering' at his disposal. Accordingly he described this wakefulness of thinking as the active mind or intellect (*nous*) which does not think anything. But precisely as *intellectus agens* it brings it about that something is taken up into thought. Thus he is obliged to say that this thought which thinks itself returns to itself only with the thinking of something else. To start out from the primacy of self-consciousness, from a form of reflection without 'light', is not to begin from a phenom-enological given. The profound consequence which must be drawn from Greek wisdom is, rather, the recognition that that form of seeing which is given over to the object is itself the genuine mode of encounter with the truth. This recognition is unambiguously contained in the word *nous* and the way in which it was used. From these reflections we can see that it was only with the trans-formation of the modern period that we began to place certainty of knowledge above everything else and, correspondingly, to accord diminished priority to phenomenological evidence. This is some-thing which has far-reaching consequences.

When Descartes's philosophical reflections led him to intro-duce the distinction between *res extensa* and *res cogitans* it sig-nified the dawning of a new epoch, the age of modern science. Both mind and body are conceived as 'substance', that is to say, neither is dependent on anything else for its existence, including *res cogitans*. It exists by virtue of the fact that it thinks itself. And it is on this basis that the whole of modern science rests. The self-certainty of self-consciousness is the unshakeable foundation of all certainty and so in the eyes of modern science of true know-ledge. This is a new, narrower sense of knowledge which first became valid in the modern period. Nietzsche was right to claim that it represents the victory of method over science. It is the reduction of truth to certainty. In the Galilean science of the seventeenth and eighteenth centuries this became the foundation for the whole vast edifice of the modern natural sciences.

Of course, on the margins of this enterprise, problems devel-oped which were to arise time and time again. The classic ex-ample is given by Leibniz. Leibniz himself describes how one day while walking in the Rosental in Leipzig he became convinced of the inevitability of Galilean physics, yet he still insisted on the indispensability of the Aristotelian conception of *entelecheia* with respect to the phenomenon of life. The things which determine our intellectual development are highly complex. For example it was the microscope – by revealing microscopic creatures and infusoria – which provided the first great confirmation of the 'animation' present in all beings, that is, the soul within them.

This was an unbelievable sensation at the time. Everything which exists was shown to possess life and soul, something which the Greeks accepted as a matter of course. Whatever is 'one' is a 'self', and it is a self because it relates to itself. Thus one of Leibniz's contemporaries, the Swabian priest Friedrich of Oetinger, defended the central significance of the concept of life, albeit in a polemic against Leibniz. Oetinger characterized the way in which animate life is present in all of its different parts under the title *sensus communis*.

This is something which was obscured by talk of the 'parts' of the soul, something which was taken over from Greek attempts to describe the latter. In order to describe its different aspects Plato had, indeed, spoken of the 'parts' of the 'soul'. But he clearly did not conceive of it – as one modern interpreter has done – as a computer which sets various different functions in operation. Aristotle quite correctly warned against taking this talk of the parts of the soul literally. The soul is not made up of parts as the body is made up of its various organs and members. As living things we are fully present in each of our different states or conditions. We are wholly taken up by anger, completely shaken by fear. We are not angry or fearful in just one part of the soul.

These insights into the ontological constitution of living beings remain as fundamental for the psychologist as they do for the doctor. An important role was also played here by Kant's recognition in the *Critique of Judgement* that we must conceive of a living thing as a unified organism, and not merely as the collective operation of exchangeable mechanical parts.

We cannot fail to recognize, then, that it is characteristic of living things always to possess this power over themselves. Kant had already brilliantly shown that no organ of the human body could be conceived merely as the means to some other end, but is always at the same time also an end in itself. Thus unity must be conceived as something differentiated. Hegel, too, with his unique speculative daring, sought to grasp the transition from life to consciousness and self-consciousness in these terms. He describes life as being something like the 'universal blood'. By this he does not simply mean the circulation of the blood which characterizes the organic unity of the higher animals, but rather the unity of life which courses through everything. This description in turn raises both the problem of the soul as something which is single, and the problem of the singularity of consciousness. To speak with Hegel: consciousness must be grasped as the unity of simplicity and infinitude. We recognize immediately that infinitude is constitutive of consciousness. We are always capable of thinking beyond things, and the reflexive structure of self-consciousness is characterized precisely by the capacity to progress through unlimited stages of reflection. It is this which constitutes self-consciousness as reflexivity.

But alongside this infinite or unlimited character, consciousness is, at the same time, unity and simplicity. That which is in consciousness is not simply sustained in the universal blood like everything else, but is rather unified in such a way that it becomes something singular for me. Here I would like to use Hegel's famous expression, 'being for itself'. By this Hegel meant that what I am aware of is at the same time something which belongs to me. It is 'for' me. I am the one who has seen it. With this a very great step is taken, the step towards language by means of which everything becomes something intended by me. Whatever I can become conscious of I make my own through the speaking and using of words. This is not the place to show how Hegel presents the transition from the stage of individual consciousness to that of 'objective spirit' or how, as a form of spirit which has become objective to us, objective spirit is no longer to be conceived of simply as the abstract thought of universality.

There is a profound saying by the Greek physician Alkmaion: 'We human beings must die because we have not learnt to connect the end with the beginning again.' What does this mean? Is the defining characteristic of human beings an intrinsic lack which we suffer in distinction to other living creatures? We are characterized by the fact that we are not simply identical with a kind of 'life' which reproduces itself, but rather that each and every one of us, as an individual, must die their own death. The individual as such is not simply part of the universal blood which finds expression in one and then another cycle of the organism, before, finally, returning to the universal cycle of nature. What this means, fundamentally, is that living beings simply constitute the species, whereas Alkmaion's saying entails the recognition that a human being is precisely not identical with the species. It is for this reason that we must die and it is why we would like to be able to believe in immortality, even though, unless we possess absolute faith in the promises of religion, we must doubt its possibility.

We saw that the wisdom of the Greeks provided confirmation of this saying of Alkmaion. But it received its most complete confirmation with the coming of Christianity, whose message of redemption from death conceived of the crucifixion of Jesus as taking the place of the suffering of death. Through the promise of resurrection the life of each individual won a predominance that it had never before possessed, and within the realm of Christian culture life and death acquired an immense importance, resisting all tendencies towards secularization. For collective ways of life other than Christianity the situation is quite different and this presents wholly new problems for the emerging global situation. These problems arise from the diversity of values ascribed to the phenomena of life and death. All these things, in turn, are closely connected with the theme of 'life and soul' and ultimately with the question concerning the immortality of the soul and the absolutely singular character of our own death. With this the soul is burdened with the strange distance from the body produced by that peculiar intimacy of one's own inner life which does not seem to leave any space for 'thoughts belonging to the shared spirit', as Hölderlin put it. We can see that the Greek belief in the soul is not really so very far removed from the experience of the modern man or woman in their everyday life situation. And here we see, too, the extent to which psychology reaches into the realm of philosophy.

12

Anxiety and Anxieties

The inner logic of language possesses a certain evidence for each of us. If we could succeed in at least partially grasping the internal connection that exists between such different things as anxiety, the various anxieties, the process of becoming anxious, the persistence of anxiety and the overcoming of anxiety, we would be in a better position to understand how anxiety can actually become an illness, whether this be termed a psychosis or described in some other way. By examining the rich spectrum of phenomena involved we can hope to discover some sort of meaning or logic lying behind them.

As a philosopher who holds Heidegger's starting point on this question to be decisive it is almost inevitable that I should place strong emphasis on his approach. For even within the discipline of psychiatry this perspective has been appropriated for the analysis of human existence. In this connection, rather against the intention of the work, Heidegger's *Being and Time* is read as a primary text of anthropology. Though Heidegger himself said that *Being and Time* contains a rich fund of anthropological insight, he never intended to make a direct contribution towards anthropology itself. Rather he wanted to give a new and expanded horizon to the question of being, which from time immemorial has characterized western philosophy as metaphysics. Heidegger's description of the phenomenon of anxiety in *Being and Time* is not intended as an anthropological account of something that one might on the whole prefer to overlook in favour of more positive states of mind. It is not a question of whether Heidegger regards human existence too negatively in holding it to be dominated by anxiety. Rather, it is people's disposition of anxiety that makes the question of the meaning of being and the meaning of nothingness visible in a new way. This is Heidegger's philosophical starting point and it is what lends the theme of anxiety such profundity and such extraordinary resonance. It is in this sense that Heidegger presents anxiety as the fundamental disposition of humankind. I am reminded of some lines by the baroque poet Logau, who shared this insight:

> Sobald ein neues Kind
> die erste Luft empfind't
> so hebt es an zu weinen.
> Die Sonne muß ihm scheinen
> den viermal zehnten Tag,
> eh als es lachen mag.
> Oh Welt, bei deinen Sachen
> ist weinen mehr als lachen.

(As soon as a newborn child feels the first touch of air it falls to crying. The sun must shine upon it for well nigh forty days before it starts to laugh. Oh in this our world, tears predominate over laughter.)

The poem points to the existence of certain fundamental phenomena which always remain present in the background and serve to characterize human beings as such. Anxiety is intimately connected with an oppressive sense of constriction, with sudden exposure to the vastness and strangeness of the world. Something of this primary experience still resides – and can still be heard – in a number of words belonging to our language. In German we find it in words such as *ungeheuer* and *unheimlich*. The word *geheuer* describes a state of being at home, of feeling safe and sound. Its negative counterpart, *ungeheuer* suggests the strange and the uncanny. When we use this word it implies that we do not feel at ease or that something does not seem quite familiar to us. *Un-geheuer* is thus a highly effective expression for the incomprehensible vastness, for the emptiness, remoteness and strangeness which takes our breath away even while we struggle to sustain our lives and to make ourselves at home in this world. The expression 'making oneself at home in the world' was a favourite one of Hegel's and he regarded it as constitutive of what it is to be human. It describes the desire to be at home with oneself, secure from any threat of danger, surrounded by a familiar, understood and understandable world where one can feel free of anxiety.

When we speak of anxiety in these terms it is clear that we are not referring to the specific phenomena with which medical anthropology is concerned but rather to something which is fundamentally constitutive of lived existence. It points to the desire to escape abroad and break open from what is oppressive and constricting. If we turn to the history of philosophy we find this idea expressed by Schelling. In his book *On the Essence of Human Freedom* Schelling writes: 'The anxiety of life drives the creature outside of its own centre.' This is like a guiding thread, an unintended commentary on our present discussion. Schelling's observation touches on the connection between what Wolfgang Blankenburg has described as the existential meaning of anxiety, as opposed to its vital or real meaning. Such anxiety carries within itself the question: why is there something rather than nothing? At the same time it raises the specific question which is the concern of the psychiatrist: how is it that anxiety in the face of life as such can develop into the various different anxieties? To some extent it is correct to say that language itself does not give us the grounds for following Kierkegaard and Heidegger in characterizing anxiety proper, as opposed to all the particular anxieties and phobias, as the fear of 'nothingness'. This characterization can only arise out of an exclusive search after the question of being. But it can also be realized by anyone who is released from the stranglehold of anxiety. Once it has receded, anxiety becomes a sort of experience of nothing, and so also of being. Heidegger has vividly described what it is that was the object of such anxiety: 'It was nothing.' If we were only able to name it, then it would already be something. It would no longer be that basic human disposition in which something which is not a thing suddenly comes upon us as the 'there' of existence. The question as to the actual meaning of this mysterious 'there', which we call wakefulness or consciousness, is therefore closely connected with the question of philosophy itself.

This 'there' represents an enigma not only for philosophy but for all of us whether we are scientifically minded or not. Heraclitus long ago recognized this truth in a number of memorable observations when he spoke of how man must kindle for himself a light in the darkness. He further describes how the state of sleep touches on that of death and how in the process of waking up we are suddenly torn from sleeping into wakefulness. Heraclitus showed moreover that the miracle of conscious life is inextricably bound up with the acceptance of death. We cannot avoid it. For man death is the self-evident counterpart to life. With this recognition we are already approaching the fundamental anthropological insight that it is characteristic of human thought to strive to grasp this mystery. As such it is something we are all familiar with. When Schelling says that the 'creature' is driven by the anxiety of life he clearly uses the term creature because he wants to refer to something more fundamental than the actual 'knowledge of death'. It is this more fundamental dimension which drives human beings to repress the thought of death. And in this connection we may recall a word which was used by Jacob Böhme, namely *Qual*, meaning agony or anguish. Böhme interpreted 'quality' as *Qual* because quality is what distinguishes one existent from another. The being of each particular thing is characterized by the isolating pain or anguish which is unique to it. It perseveres in being in its own special way, gives itself form and so unfolds its own particular quality.

These remarks confirm in an important way the fact that anxiety concerning death is indeed a phenomenon which not only psychologists and psychiatrists but ultimately every observer is able to describe. It is only an intensification of that anxiety which is part of the fundamental disposition of human beings. It is because we are thinking beings that we must concern ourselves with death. This is an ancient article of human knowledge.

In this connection I am particularly interested in Aeschylus' profound drama, *Prometheus Bound*. I can still remember from my childhood a small sculpture which stood on the piano in my parents' house, a bronze Prometheus with a silver eagle feeding on his liver. It represented the famous story of the suffering and chained Prometheus which is retold in dramatic form by Aeschylus. The myth relates how Prometheus stole fire from heaven and taught mankind to work with it. But Aeschylus presents the story in a way which makes the theft of fire almost incidental. Prometheus glories in having performed the greatest possible service to man – who had been left so poor and defenceless by Zeus – by depriving him of the knowledge of his own death. This was Prometheus' real gift. Previously man had lived in a state of gloom and idleness, awaiting death, dwelling in caves, just like many other creatures. But once the knowledge of the hour of his death was taken away from him hope rose up and with it the first great human desire to transform the world into a habitable place. Aeschylus depicts Prometheus boasting how through his theft of fire he has brought about all of man's great skills and above all the *sophia*, or wisdom, involved in human crafts. The profundity of Aeschylus' interpretation lies in the way he suggests that it was precisely the development of these skills which enabled mankind to conceal from himself and so to forget the fact of death, whereas the original myth of the theft of fire had been interpreted only in terms of the discovery of the skills and crafts alone. Plato took a further step of interpretation. He has Protagoras express the idea that man's inventive spirit was first awoken through the possession of fire. But Plato goes on to describe the significance of this great new gift in terms of number, which lies between indeterminacy and unity. And for Plato this also implies the realm of dialectics, that is, of philosophy itself.

But the interpretation brought by Aeschylus to the ancient myth is already a very profound one I think. It is an astonishing thought: the knowledge of one's own death transforms what is characteristic of man, namely the capacity to anticipate the future, into its very opposite, into the dull endurance of a cave-bound exist-ence. But this myth signifies the forgetting of death so that he no longer has to reckon with it. And yet, since no reckoning with death is possible and since death can never be overcome, this forgetting of death is never a real forgetting or overcoming, but rather constitutes life itself. Thus the whole investigative genius of man presses forward into an incalculable future, or rather, be-yond every calculable and incalculable future into the experience of transcendence.

What all this actually shows is how the anxiety of life, which wrests mankind from the rest of nature, has given human beings a certain distance from things. As the Greeks say, it is through the *logos*, through the possession of language, that a person is able to think something and at the same time hold certain pos-sibilities open. The anthropological basis of anxiety testifies to a specifically human characteristic, that is, that a person has a dis-tance from their own self. Heidegger saw in this the inauthenticity of an existence permanently absorbed in life, and contrasted it with authentic existence which is prepared to face anxiety. But this inauthenticity also belongs to human nature.

What we can immediately grasp from all this is the connection between anxiety and the various specific anxieties or phobias. The Greek word *phobos* is generally translated as 'fear', but it is actually more closely connected with 'horror'. For the Greek word literally means that something makes one's hair stand on end and the Greeks conceived it in just such an immediately vivid and physical way. But whether we use the term phobias or anxieties, language only gives us a first indication which must be pursued by developing a more considered distinction. We need to go be-yond what language tells us, and for this reason Heidegger spoke of 'care'. All care, all solicitude, is care for or about something, just as all anxiety is anxiety in the face of something or anxiety about something. However, precisely the plurality of anxieties refers us back to the fundamental disposition of human beings. Humankind has completely emerged from the condition of being instinctually determined through and through and it is this which distinguishes humans from the other highly developed animals.

Let us consider why it is that we can observe ever increasing anxiety in the world today. In my opinion, the particular form of knowledge and certainty which modern science produces through experiment and prediction has increased the human need for security. There is a well-known sociological expression for this form of knowledge which was, I believe, first introduced by Max Scheler: *Herrschaftswissen*, that is, a controlling or mastering knowledge. This is not a bad expression. All doctors will admit that they quite naturally talk about 'mastering something'. Of course, they are also aware of the limits of such mastery and this is something they must also resign themselves to in their everyday medical practice. None the less it is clear that the need for security is intimately bound up with this knowledge which promises mastery and control.

The transition to the modern period received its classic formulation in the work of Descartes and in the concept of method. We are 'certain' of the things we know. On those occasions when I have the opportunity of conversing with people working in the field of natural science this becomes abundantly clear: for such scientists what exists are *facts*! This sounds impressive and intimidating. However, as philosophers we must ask what facts are and reflect, for instance, on the example of statistics, which teaches us the ambiguity of all claims concerning the existence of facts. Despite all the progress which has been made through the most recent attempts at mastering the neurological phenomena of anxiety, it still remains beyond doubt that anxiety concerning existence is something which belongs inseparably to the life and nature of human beings. In earlier times this was experienced as the anxiety felt in the presence of storms and the violence of the elements. Although we no longer feel such anxiety today, there is none the less an anxiety peculiar to modern civilization. This, too, is something atmospheric; we say that it is 'in the air'. We can ask whether it is the need for security in our lives which lies behind this feeling. Here we need only consider the example of the political realm, where people act as though they could completely exclude anxiety and everything connected with the process of being and becoming anxious. This argument is used quite consciously in certain political situations where a decision must be made to reduce public disquiet.

But this intensified need for security is, of course, not everything. The fundamental question which lies behind this need concerns the answers we must provide to the fundamental human disposition of anxiety in life. We build our lives within the realm of 'care' in so far as we constantly concern ourselves with different things, constantly try to procure them, constantly live in a state of concern. As I see it, this is how we make ourselves at home in the world we create. But today this presents us with particular difficulties because the future seems so devoid of hope. Without doubt, over thousands of years of human history, the various religions have successfully provided a framework for the attempt to make ourselves at home in this way. They presented, as it were, forms of objectification that offered protection against the anxiety of existence which people – those peculiar thinking and questioning beings who are never wholly one with nature – find placed on them. We live under a constant threat which is clearly inseparable from life itself. Logau has described how this feeling of being threatened is vividly articulated in the cry of the newborn child. Yet the anxiety which is part of today's civilization expresses the fact that we experience this threat as something nameless, and thus as something which is increasingly difficult to grasp. We no longer know what it is that so clearly seems to govern the entire order of our existence and yet seems quite independent of our own actions. My predecessor in Heidelberg, Karl Jaspers, named our epoch the age of anonymous responsibility. For indeed we can no longer say either who is responsible or who it is that we are supposed to be responsible to. None of us can properly be described as responsible. In today's highly complex and thoroughly organized society no one is in a position to believe they can completely master the problems which cause concern and anxiety in our civilization.

Yet there is something else which is important here. Modern science has contributed to the dissolution of the various religions and so created a vacuum. This can clearly be seen from the few utopian attempts to organize the social and political order in a supposedly 'scientific' manner, something whose breakdown we are witnessing today. But there is a third phenomenon which has already played an important role in the context of our discussion: to what extent can human life endure truth at all? This is a question which Nietzsche formulated and it represents one of the provocative challenges which his thought poses for our epoch with ever greater force. In his despair at the inability of the Enlightenment and of modern science to answer the most fundamental human questions, Nietzsche arrived at his provocative doctrine of the 'eternal return of the same'. He was a great moralist and with this doctrine he wanted to show how in the face of absolute hopelessness we must learn to be resolute. What he demanded of us was genuine morality, something more than human: 'I teach you the overman.'

With these reflections and explanations I have attempted to call to mind the connection that exists between fundamental anxiety as our fundamental disposition and all the anxieties which in their different forms constitute our lived existence. This should now enable us to address the question as to what illness means in the context of anxiety. It is quite rightly said that anxiety is not itself an illness. Yet there are psychoses, indeed anxiety psychoses, where anxiety apparently becomes an illness or at least appears in the form of an illness. What is the connection here? I speak, of course, as a layman. One of the advantages or rather pieces of good fortune which I have enjoyed in my life is that my contact with the doctor has almost always been as a friend and rarely as a patient. If we attempt to discover the real difference between illness and health, then we must recognize that illness cannot be defined by the contrast with a notion of health which is in turn derived from the establishment of standard values. There are so many marginal factors which cannot be measured that the results deriving entirely from what can be measured lose their significance by comparision. The picture of the individual which is constructed on the basis of standard values is an extremely precarious and unreliable one. It is only when we start out from the recognition that the distinction between health and illness cannot be so clearly defined that we can remind ourselves that even today medical interns must still begin by asking patients in what way they are feeling unwell. This is something I have observed on each of the few occasions when I have required the services of a doctor as a doctor. That the intern must ask this question shows that the physical organism is conscious of itself and capable of telling us about its general condition. This can protect us from the danger of becoming ill through the imposition of standard values.

What should the perspective of the psychiatrist be on such matters? We are concerned here with a typical question asked by interns. Yet a large proportion of so-called mental illnesses rest on the fact that this feeling of being unwell is not consciously present or is at least consistently and firmly denied. It is also one of the great problems in psychoanalysis that only patients who are already aware that they are unwell can take the decisive step towards analysis. As far as I know, no analyst would accept someone as a patient who had been compelled to enter into treatment. It is a patient's own acute awareness of illness combined with their sense of distress which, as it were, compels them in the first place to turn for help to a doctor or an analyst. But we must ask what illness 'really' is and try to recognize how it is located on the continuum between the flexibility with which we normally deal with our daily worries and concerns and what happens when we fall outside of the normal pattern of caring for and looking after ourselves.

This is something which we can compare with the phenomenon of equilibrium. You will all remember – I, at least, have not forgotten it from my childhood – what it was like trying to learn to ride a bicycle. What is astonishing about this experience is that as soon as one learns to do it properly it immediately seems so much easier than it did when one still had to hold tightly on to the handlebars with the greatest effort. Suddenly one gains a sense of equilibrium and then it is as if everything simply goes by itself, as we can see with those young people who are able to speed by with folded arms. This image should serve to make it clear that this sliding scale of effort and relaxation is a quite natural part of human life. For this reason I consider the employment of average values in medicine and in doctors' practices to have a dangerous side to it. In any case, it is clear that there is a broad range of variable factors here. What I am fundamentally concerned with is the nature of this scale of changes and where the points of continuity and of breakdown are to be located. For we do possess an extraordinary flexibility in regard to everything that we do and everything that affects us. How is it, then, that this flexibility can break down? I want to claim that this question cannot be answered through any merely objective strategy of questioning and research. The distinction between health and illness is a pragmatic one and the only person who has access to it is the actual person who is feeling ill, the person who can no longer cope with all the demands of life and so decides to go to the doctor. Finally, therefore, it seems to me that we must recognize and accept the fundamental disposition of anxiety in the face of life, and equally of death; this is what Romano Guardini has described as the ontological privilege of mankind. The life which awakens to thinking and questioning thinks and questions beyond all limits. To know anxiety and to be unable to grasp death, this is the human birth cry which never wholly dies away.

13

Hermeneutics and Psychiatry

From time immemorial psychiatry has occupied a unique position within the sphere of medical science and the healing arts in general, just as medicine has always occupied a unique position in relation to the other sciences. As an art of medicine, psychiatry always lies on the borderline of science, drawing life from its indissoluble connection with 'praxis'. Praxis, however, is not merely an application of scientific knowledge. Rather, aspects of praxis react back on research, and the results of research must consistently prove and confirm themselves in turn with reference to praxis. There are, then, good reasons why doctors do not see their profession as equivalent either to that of the scientist or researcher, or to that of a mere technician, who would simply 'apply' scientific knowledge and discoveries with the purpose of restoring health. Part of what a doctor does closely resembles an art, and is something which cannot be conveyed through theoretical instruction. It is this which it is appropriate to call the 'art of healing'.

Praxis is more than the mere application of knowledge. And 'practice' refers to the complete sphere of life of the medical profession, and not simply to 'the practice' as one specific workplace among others in the whole world of work. Praxis possesses its own unique world. Something similar is the case with jurisprudence, which has always been aware of its unique status. Even in the age of science, it hesitated a long time before taking on the title of a legal science and thereby separating itself from its authentic character as prudence, the exercise of legal insight and the art of law. With jurisprudence, too, praxis is inseparable from science. And here, too, the legal profession has had to build up its own clientele with effort and, indeed, against popular resistance to legal shysters and the manipulation of the law. Likewise, from the very beginning the art of medicine has always needed to justify itself.

The relationship between the doctor and the patient, however, is different in kind. Especially in the age of science, which is our own age, it is the other technical aspect of the doctor's profession which has prompted ever-renewed reflection. Above all, it is the patients approaching the doctor for help who are so seduced by the astonishing technical means of modern medicine that they see nothing but this aspect and marvel only at the doctor's scientific competence. A patient's own state of need encourages this tendency to privilege the technical wonders of modern medicine above everything else and to forget that the application of this knowledge is a highly demanding and responsible task of the broadest human and social dimensions.

If it is only with some hesitation that doctors in general can be classified as natural scientists, this is especially the case with psychiatrists. The science and praxis of psychiatry are always to be found on the narrow borderline between the knowledge domain of the natural sciences with their attempt to understand nature by rational means, and recognition of the enigmatic character of mental and psychological problems. For the human being is not only a natural object. Rather, each of us is, in a mysterious way, unknown both to ourselves and to others. As a public person, as a neighbour, in the family and at work, each one of us responds to innumerable and incalculable effects and influences, burdens and problems. There are always unpredictable elements which play their part. The things which require understanding here are quite different from those laws of nature which highly developed research techniques are increasingly able to reveal and explain.

The concern with things which are not understood, the attempt to grasp the unpredictable character of the spiritual and mental life of human beings, is the task of the art of understanding which we call hermeneutics. In earlier centuries this learned Greek word could be used to describe our knowledge of humankind in general. And this was also true when the limits of the new science of the seventeenth and eighteenth centuries began to reveal themselves and when, in the age of Goethe and the Romantics, it was realized that each of us represents a profound enigma, both to ourselves and to others.

It is clear that the art of understanding plays an important role in many different domains of knowledge. Its significance for biblical interpretation and pastoral work, for jurisprudence and the interpretation of the law, has long been known. Understanding plays a role wherever rules cannot simply be applied, and this includes the entire sphere of collective human life. Thus it transpires that we can prove incomprehensible to ourselves, that we can fail to understand ourselves, just as we can fail to understand others. To this extent it is not surprising that precisely in the age of science philosophy began to recognize and appreciate the limits of following rules and of the new possibilities opened up by science.

If our century really has taken a new step in philosophical thinking, then it lies in the realization that it is not only reason and thought which stand at the centre of philosophy but also language itself, the means through which everything comes to expression. In the age of science it is not so astonishing that, for over a century now, language, like everything else, should have been considered in terms of its potential mastery and utility. This has meant that language was thematized as a world of signs, with the model being provided by the scientific success of the symbolic languages which had been developed out of mathematics. Thus it was that philosophy came to be guided by the ideal of an unambiguous artificial language which could overcome all *idola fori* ('the idols of the marketplace') through the unambiguous expression of meaning. Ever since Leibniz and the eighteenth century, one of the highest goals has been represented by the thought that mathematical logic might ultimately be refined into an ideal of unambiguous description, thus turning philosophy at last into a true science. In the meantime, however, and quite in the contrary direction, we have come to recognize the productive diversity of human languages and their embeddedness in contexts of human action. Even the constructivist ideal of a generative grammar has itself incorporated the principle of creativity. The development of such grammars represent fascinating achievements of insight and logic. Admittedly, however, they limit themselves to the formal and the functional dimensions, without regard for the rich wealth of content which is expressed through language. In what is called analytic philosophy, for example, the different dimensions of speech are only covered from a particular aspect. And something similar is the case with the extremely interesting insights into the implicit grammar of the mythical imagination which have been developed by Claude Lévi-Strauss and the structuralists. These too are fascinating contributions to our general enlightenment, and yet they cannot replace the mysterious insight vouchsafed by the world of myth.

Natural language contains other intimations and harbours other secrets which are not exhausted by the astonishing function of linguistic communication which can, and has been, replaced by artificial codes. There is yet another form of communality in which a language, as our mother tongue, binds us together in the exercise of our thought and in the application of our reason. The capacity to speak is not simply a natural gift which enables us to communicate with each other in the same way as artificial sign systems do. Rather, thanks to the possession of language, human society is wholly different in range and character from the society of animals, 'since a dialogue is what we are, being able listen to one another,' as Hölderlin expresses it. The entire formation of our life-world through the construction of an ethical order, as well as the development of religious and cultural traditions, can be traced back to the ultimate miracle of language. This does not consist in the ability to signal to one another, in order to regulate the behaviour of the species, but in the ability to form a particular language community and thereby a common world. What is new is the ability to listen to one another, the capacity to attend to another human being. Herein consists the universal dimension of hermeneutics, a dimension which encompasses and supports all of our reason and thought. It is for this reason that hermeneutics is not an ancillary discipline, serving merely to provide an important methodological framework for various other sciences. Rather, it extends into the heart of philosophy, which is not only the study of logical thinking and the method of inquiry, but a pursuit of the logic of dialogue.

Thinking is the dialogue of the soul with itself. This is how Plato described thinking, and this means at the same time that thinking is listening to the answers that we give ourselves, and that are given to us, when we raise the question of the incomprehensible. To understand the incomprehensible, above all to understand that which requires to be understood, this is common to all the different forms of reflection contained in the religions, in the art of different peoples, and in the light cast by our own historical tradition. Here there are always new questions, and with every answer a new question is raised. This is hermeneutics as philosophy.

Once the task of hermeneutics is seen in this way, the proximity of hermeneutics to psychiatry becomes clear. If philosophy is an attempt to understand the incomprehensible, an attempt to take up the major human questions to which the religions, the world of myth, poetry, art and culture all offer responses, then it must encompass the mystery of the beginning and the end, of being and nothing, of birth and death, and, above all, of good and evil. These are enigmatic questions which do not appear to have any answer that would constitute 'knowledge'. Psychiatrists will immediately recognize how particularly exposed they are to such unexplained phenomena, which they encounter in the emotional disturbances and mental illness they are required to treat. The psychiatrist is familiar with religious mania and its often murderous or suicidal force, which can drive the individual or a whole group or sect to its death. The psychiatrist is also familiar with forms of obsessive love which can lead to total ruin. To the psychiatrist as a scientifically enlightened individual all these forms of obsession are well known. Whether understood as possession by demons who must be driven out, as divine inspiration, or as delusions such as those pursuing the raging Ajax or Orestes across the Greek stage – 'I am of the race of Tantalus' – they are all recognizable to the modern enlightened person. The doctor who is aware of such afflictions and encounters them in the concrete forms of mythic witness, the art of poetry or tragic mimesis may not always know how to translate what is being expressed through works of art into the language of science. Perhaps the more likely reaction is the one illustrated in the classic case of the doctor in the audience of the first performance of Gerhart Hauptmann's *Vor Sonnenaufgang* at the end of the last century. When the cries of a long and protracted birth came from the back of the stage and continued painfully to dominate the scene, the doctor indignantly threw a pair of forceps on to the set.

Whether on the stage or in the experience of professional life, the psychiatrist encounters uncanny and incomprehensible phenomena, and interprets madness as a form of emotional disturbance and mental illness. But for the psychiatrist the category of illness, which I use here as if it were self-explanatory, is not simply given in the same way as it is for other forms of medical diagnosis. Normally it is the case that the doctor puts forward a diagnosis when the patient comes to the doctor complaining of not feeling well, that something is 'lacking'. The patient defines health and illness in terms of this lack of something, even if it turns out to be the case that nothing is really lacking at all. In general it is this recognition that he or she is ill – even where it is misplaced – that leads the patient to go the doctor. But the psychiatrist must deal above all with cases where the patient's insight into their own illness is disturbed, and even, as with the hypochondriac or someone who simulates an illness, with cases in which all possibility of reaching understanding seems to have been removed. Here the hermeneutic task of the psychiatrist diverges significantly from the· one normally involved in the medical treatment of a patient, including the forging of a human partnership, no matter how fleeting, between doctor and patient. Here the possibility of forming such a partnership seems to be excluded. Even questions concerning the borderline area of psychosomatic illness are generally met with resistance by the patient, who thereby seeks to protect the work of the unconscious. Here the specific hermeneutic problem of psychiatry, so familiar to the psychiatrist, is once again revealed. The psychiatrist must seek to reach understanding with the patient, even where the patient withdraws from such understanding. We can find further confirmation for this when we consider that it is an indispensable precondition of the psychoanalytic 'talking cure' that patients enter into analysis on the basis of their own recognition that they are unwell.

In recent decades, above all through the work of Michel Foucault, the concept of mental illness and abnormality has once again become a problem from the social and political point of view. It cannot be denied that an awareness of social norms, as well as corresponding forms of behaviour on the part of society as a whole, always contribute to the definition of such a concept of illness, and so render it problematic. Social scientists and philosophers recognize this problem under the heading 'genius and madness'. It is precisely with artists and the creatively gifted who live on the edges of society that we encounter a form of 'abnormality' which makes such a rigid construction of categories difficult. Thus in many problematic cases the whole language of madness has been contested, though perhaps more by those involved in the discussion of cultural life than by doctors. In Germany we have the case of the poet Friedrich Hölderlin. In light of the eclipse of his faculties at the end of his life, a large number of Hölderlin's poetic works appeared so incomprehensible and eccentric to his contemporaries that even his friends, when they set about producing subsequent editions of his work, deliberately omitted many of his most important poems. Thus it is that an important part of Hölderlin's poetic output, which belongs to his mature years before his complete psychological withdrawal, was only rediscovered in this century. Like a true contemporary he has inspired the poetic writing of our time. Even the poems from the very last years, from the time when he was undoubtedly suffering from an all-consuming mental illness, have subsequently proved to be epoch-making.

The alternative which is discussed by modern scholarship as to whether Hölderlin was suffering from a genuine or a simulated mental illness must ultimately be seen as setting up a false question. Someone can also move from simulated to genuine illness, as is shown by the case of Pirandello's Henry IV. Nor are things so very different in the case of Friedrich Nietzsche. Here it is not so much his illness that is in question but how it came to arise and what caused it. And this only intensifies the difficulties involved in separating out what belongs to his madness and what is truly significant in his later writings, a task which invites ever new interpretations and solutions. Is it still something we can understand or rather something incomprehensible when Nietzsche signs himself as 'Dionysus or the crucified one'? The concept of comprehensibility proves itself to be extremely vague. In the case of psychoanalysis, too, which seeks to gather together some sort of meaning from out of the fragments of the patient's dream-life, the concept of comprehensibility begins to blur and become hazy. In having to provide expertise in the making of decisions about a patient's mental well-being, the psychiatrist knows from everyday practice the difficulties involved in establishing such borderlines. And before a court of law, where it is a question of establishing someone's soundness of mind and so their responsibility in the face of the law, this becomes a pressure which can weigh on the psychiatrist's conscience. Equally, the spread of drug-related illnesses and addiction should serve to make us even more aware of the almost insoluble difficulties involved in establishing at what point the transition is made from divine madness, obsessive love, jealousy, hate and friendship to the limits of responsibility and soundness of mind.

However, the outlook of modern psychiatrists who have at their disposal infinitely subtle instruments for the measurement and collection of data is dominated by a completely different and massive set of objectifications as regards both the effects of illness and the discovery of the correct means for treating such effects. From this perspective the limit cases we have been discussing will appear as no more than marginal phenomena. However, the fact that doctors have recourse to various possibilities for mastering an illness, such as the resources of modern pharmaceutics, does not make the uncanny obscurity surrounding mental illness any less incomprehensible. In many such cases the partnership between doctor and patient remains separated by an unbridgeable divide. Here it seems that no hermeneutics can help to bridge this gap, and yet even in these most difficult cases the doctor – and, who knows, perhaps the patient as well – must give due recognition to the fact that what is involved is always a relationship between two human beings.

Albert Camus once related the following story. In a psychiatric hospital a passing doctor noticed one of his patients fishing with a rod in a bathtub. As he walked by, mindful of this indispensable partnership between two human beings, the doctor asked the patient: 'Are they biting?' To which the patient replied: 'Idiot. Can't you even see that it is a bathtub?' How all the different threads interweave here! In the midst of the most complete delusion – there is clarity. What an unbridgeable distance from the genial condescension intended in the doctor's jest! And what a sudden fall for the doctor! Who is the idiot here? To some extent we all feel ourselves to be the idiot when someone fails to understand a joke or takes something literally which was meant ironically. And yet the doctor must at least try to forge some sort of connection with the patient through whatever fragments of sense he can grasp hold of. The doctor attempts to understand the patient's mania for fishing and its fascination, and, at least in humour, seeks to participate in the power of illusion which governs it, thereby seeking at least to participate in something. The patient's response is merciless. The force of his madness is so strong that he regards the doctor as an ignoramus, as must always be the case with those who do not share and believe in his delusions. This story rather wonderfully reveals how dangerous it is to try to participate in the delusions of someone who is so disturbed, and how there is a permanent risk of becoming entangled there. It discloses the uncanny character of the abyss that separates us from the mentally disturbed patient. For the patient, the superiority of the doctor is nothing but ignorance. In order to defend his fixed ideas, the patient's resistance makes the one who possesses knowledge into the one who is ignorant.

Ultimately this should not surprise us. Such a rigid concept as that of total incomprehensibility – one in which all attempts to understand necessarily fail – seems almost inappropriate for describing realms of human life. For our concepts of sickness and health also essentially describe vital phenomena, that flux of life whose ebb and flow accompany our very sense of being. In order to do justice to this, both in the realm of diagnosis and of treatment, the doctor needs more than just scientific and technical knowledge and professional experience. Of course, the doctor will bring into play all the instruments available to hospitals and modern medicine in order to make an informed diagnosis based on the objective results of tests and examinations. The doctor will also freely be prepared to allow standard values to guide the assessment of results, so that certain deviations will appear temporarily or wholly unimportant. Such a diagnosis will be irreproachable if nothing too unusual is the case. But this is not everything.

I knew a famous pathologist who on one occasion said to me: 'When I am ill I go to my colleague who is an intern' – who was also a famous man – 'and ask him to tell me what the problem is. Then I seek out a doctor who can treat me.' Of course, treatment too has its own rules and prescriptions. But with a good doctor all sorts of other factors come into play, and these allow the treatment to develop into what is ultimately an individual partnership between the doctor and the patient. Its successful end should be the release of the patient, and the patient's return to their everyday life. When it is a matter of a chronic illness, or of a hopeless case when no recovery can be expected, then the doctor's concern must be to lessen the patient's suffering. Here the contribution of those factors which cannot be objectified is even more important. The doctor is burdened with terrible problems, especially in treating the dying. To what extent may the doctor seek to ease the patient's suffering when what is thereby taken away is not only the patient's pain but also their 'person', their freedom and responsibility for their own life, and ultimately even awareness of their own death?

Our reflections on the role of hermeneutics in psychiatry have once again taken us far beyond the boundaries of this vast discipline. From the standpoint of the doctor, too, the psychophysical unity of man cannot be denied. Is it such a bad thing for a convention of psychiatrists to become aware of the universality of hermeneutics? Such an awareness would help psychiatrists to realize that the science of psychiatry is not just one particularly comprehensive special science within the sphere of medical art and science, whose increasing technical abilities so inspire our admiration. Moreover, psychiatrists will come to recognize that the borderlines between such specialized disciplines cannot really be strictly drawn. The 'soul' does not represent just one particular domain among others, but rather reflects the totality of the embodied existence of the human being. This is something which Aristotle knew. The soul is the living power of the body itself.

Index

Index by Linda English

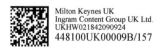
Milton Keynes UK
Ingram Content Group UK Ltd.
UKHW021842090924
448100UK00009B/157